BARIATRIC DIET 2024

110 Menu Recipes to Support Your Weight Loss Journey Nutritional Strategies and Practical Advice for a New Life

TERY LONG

DISCLAIMER

Please note that the content of this book is based on personal experience and various sources of information. This book aims to provide useful and informative material on the topics covered in the publication. It is sold with the understanding that the author and publisher are not engaged in rendering any personal medical, health care, or other professional services in the book. The reader should consult his or her physician, health care provider, or other competent professional before adopting any suggestions in this book or drawing any conclusions. The author and publisher expressly disclaim any responsibility for any liability, loss, or risk, personal or otherwise, arising, directly or indirectly, from the use and application of any contents of this book.

NOTE

In the context of this book, when we refer to "a cup" as a unit of measurement for ingredients, we mean using a standard kitchen cup with a capacity of approximately 2 milliliters. It is essential to use a measuring cup to get the right quantities of ingredients. If you don't have a measuring cup, you can use a graduated measuring cup, making sure to correctly correspond to the proportions indicated. Here are some examples 1 Cup of flour 100 gr. 1 cup of rice 200 gr. 1 Cup of Quinoa 200 g, It is recommended to level the dry ingredients in the cup using a spatula or the blade of a knife to obtain an accurate measurement. For liquid ingredients it is recommended to fill the cup to the brim without squeezing or leaving gaps.

TABLE OF CONTENT

RECIPES APPETIZERS AND SMOOTHIE

RECIPES FIRST DISHES

RECIPES SECOND DISHES

INTRODUCTION WHAT IS THE BARIATRIC DIET

The bariatric diet is an eating regimen specifically designed for people who have had bariatric surgery, such as gastric bypass, sleeve gastrectomy, or gastric banding. This diet is critical to ensuring the long-term success of the surgery and to helping patients achieve and maintain significant weight loss. Goals of the Bariatric Diet: 1. Post-Operative Healing: In the first days and weeks after surgery, the diet is geared towards promoting healing of the stomach and intestines. In this phase, you mainly consume clear liquids and soft foods. 2. Reduction of Calorie Intake: In the long term, the bariatric diet aims to significantly reduce your daily calorie intake, while still ensuring you get all essential nutrients.

3. Prevention of Nutritional Deficiencies: Due to alterations in digestion and absorption of nutrients, it is essential to follow a balanced dietary plan and often supplement vitamins and minerals. 4. Weight Management: The diet helps patients maintain the weight loss achieved with surgery and prevent weight regain. Key Principles of the Bariatric Diet: Small Portions: Because the stomach is significantly smaller, portions should be much smaller than pre-op. Slow and Thorough Chewing: It is crucial to chew your food very well to aid digestion and prevent problems such as blockages. High Protein Intake: Protein is essential for maintaining muscle mass and supporting metabolism. –

Limiting Sugars and Fats: Foods rich in sugars and fats can cause unpleasant symptoms such as "dumping syndrome", characterized by nausea, diarrhea and abdominal cramps. Evolution of the Diet: The bariatric diet evolves in different phases, ranging from an immediate postoperative liquid diet to a well-balanced solid diet. Each phase is designed to adapt to the healing process and the patient's new digestive abilities. In summary, the bariatric diet is a crucial element for the success of bariatric surgery. Following this eating plan carefully helps optimize the results of your surgery and maintain optimal long-term health.

OBJECTIVES OF THE BARIATRIC DIET

The bariatric diet is designed to support and optimize the results of bariatric surgery, with a specific focus on several crucial goals: 1. Support Postoperative Healing: In the first days and weeks after surgery, the primary goal is to promote healing of the stomach and intestines. During this phase, the diet consists mainly of clear liquids and soft foods, to avoid stress on the digestive system. 2. Facilitate Weight Loss: One of the main goals of the bariatric diet is to promote significant weight loss by dramatically reducing calorie intake and improving the body's metabolic efficiency. 3. Prevent Nutritional Deficiencies: After bariatric surgery, the body may have difficulty absorbing some essential nutrients. The diet is therefore structured for ensure an adequate intake of vitamins, minerals and proteins, often accompanied by the use of supplements. 4. Maintain Muscle Mass: Another goal is to preserve muscle mass during weight loss. This is achieved through a high protein intake and adequate physical activity, to prevent the body from using muscle tissue as an energy source. 5. Prevent Post-Operative Complications: The diet is also aimed at minimizing the risk of complications such as "dumping syndrome", which can occur when foods rich in sugar or fat are consumed too quickly. To avoid these complications, the diet limits these types of foods and encourages slow, controlled consumption. 6. Promote Sustainable Eating Habits: The bariatric diet is not just a temporary plan, but aims to establish long-term healthy and sustainable eating habits. This includes eating smaller portions, choosing nutritious foods and adopting a regular meal routine. 7. Support Psychological and Emotional Wellbeing: In addition to the physical aspects, the bariatric diet also takes into account the patient's psychological well-being. Adapting to a new way of eating can be an emotional challenge, so the diet often includes psychological support to manage lifestyle changes. In summary, the bariatric diet is designed to be a pillar in the postsurgical weight loss journey, promoting effective healing, safe and lasting weight loss, and an overall improvement in the patient's quality of life.

PHASES OF THE BARIATRIC DIET

The bariatric diet is divided into different phases, which gradually evolve to adapt to the patient's recovery and new digestive needs. Each phase has specific goals and gradually introduces more solid foods, while ensuring that the patient receives the necessary nutrients without overloading the digestive system. 1. Phase 1: Clear Liquid Diet (First 12 Days) Objective: Promote immediate healing of the stomach and reduce the risk of complications. Allowed Foods: Water, clear broth, sugar-free gelatin, sugar-free herbal teas, sugar-free popsicles. Characteristics: This phase typically lasts one or two days after surgery. The patient should sip liquids slowly and drink small amounts frequently to avoid nausea and discomfort.

2. Phase 2: Complete Liquid Diet (37 Days) Goal: Begin providing nutrition while continuing to protect the stomach. Allowed foods: Vegetable milks, protein shakes, low-fat and smooth yogurt, cream broths, diluted fruit juices, liquid protein supplements. Characteristics: During this phase, the patient can introduce thicker and more nutritious liquids, focusing mainly on protein and liquid intake to maintain hydration. **3. Phase 3: Puree Diet (24 Weeks)** Goal: Reintroduce solid foods in a highly digestible form. Allowed foods: Pureed foods such as fruit and vegetable purees, pureed fish and lean meat, scrambled eggs, tofu, Greek yogurt, pureed legumes. Characteristics: Foods at this stage must have a smooth, mushy consistency. The portions are very small, and the patient must continue to eat slowly and chew well.

4. Phase 4: Semisolid Diet (46 Weeks) Objective: To accustom the stomach to more solid foods while maintaining adequate protein intake. Allowed Foods: Soft, easy-to-chew foods such as chicken, fish, cooked vegetables, well-cooked cereals, cottage cheese, low-fat cheeses. Characteristics: Food must be soft and easily chewable. This phase gradually prepares the patient for the reintroduction of a more normal diet. **5. Phase 5: Solid Diet (6 Weeks Onwards)** Objective: Achieve a balanced and sustainable diet in the long term. Allowed Foods: All foods, with some exceptions. It is important to continue to avoid foods high in sugar, fat and refined carbohydrates. Focus on lean proteins, vegetables, low-sugar fruits and whole grains. Characteristics: This phase represents the transition to a normal diet, with very small portions and a continuous focus on careful chewing and slow consumption. The diet must be balanced, rich in proteins, fiber and essential nutrients. 6. Long-Term Maintenance Goal: Stabilize weight and maintain a healthy lifestyle. Allowed Foods: A balanced diet similar to Phase 5, with occasional adjustments to avoid weight gain. Features: Patients should continue to follow a dietary plan that supports weight maintenance and prevention of nutritional deficiencies, with continued emphasis on protein, hydration and portion control. These steps are critical to ensuring the success of bariatric surgery and helping patients develop healthy eating habits that will last a lifetime.

WEEKLY MENU

Sample Weekly Menu for the Bariatric Diet (Solid Phase) This sample weekly menu is designed for the solid phase of the bariatric diet, which begins approximately 6 weeks after surgery. It is important to note that portions must be very small, and the patient must eat slowly, chewing each bite well. Monday Breakfast: 1 hard-boiled egg 1 tablespoon of low-fat ricotta 1 slice of avocado Snack: 1 low-fat Greek yogurt Lunch: 60g of grilled chicken breast 2 tablespoons of pureed carrots Snack: 1 small piece of low-fat cheese Dinner: 60g of fish fillet steamed 2 tablespoons of cooked vegetables (courgettes or spinach) Tuesday Breakfast: 1 tablespoon of cottage cheese 1 tablespoon of cut strawberries Snack: 1 hard-boiled egg Lunch: 60g of roast turkey 2 tablespoons of cauliflower puree Snack: 1 small piece of low-fat cheese Dinner: 60g baked fish with herbs 2 tablespoons steamed broccoli Wednesday Breakfast:

1 scrambled egg 1 tablespoon cooked spinach Snack: 1 low-fat Greek yogurt Lunch: 60g grilled lean beef fillet 2 tablespoons pumpkin puree Snack: 1/2 apple without peel Dinner: 60g roast chicken 2 tablespoons mashed potatoes desserts Thursday Breakfast: 1 hard-boiled egg 1 slice of avocado Snack: 1 tablespoon of low-fat ricotta Lunch: 60g of steamed salmon fillet 2 tablespoons of steamed green beans Snack: 1 small piece of low-fat cheese Dinner: 60g of chopped turkey meat, cooked with vegetables 2 tablespoons of carrot puree Friday Breakfast: 1 tablespoon of cottage cheese 1 tablespoon of blueberries Snack: 1 hard-boiled egg Lunch: 60g of baked white fish 2 tablespoons of broccoli puree Snack: 1 low-fat Greek yogurt Dinner: 60g of grilled chicken 2 tablespoons mashed sweet potatoes Saturday Breakfast: 1 scrambled egg 1 slice of tomato Snack: 1 tablespoon low-fat ricotta Lunch: 60g lean pork fillet 2 tablespoons mashed cauliflower Snack: 1/2 pear without peel

Dinner: 60g of steamed swordfish 2 tablespoons of cooked spinach Sunday Breakfast: 1 hard-boiled egg 1 tablespoon of cottage cheese Snack: 1 low-fat Greek yogurt Lunch: 60g of baked chicken fillet 2 tablespoons of pumpkin puree Snack: 1 small piece of low-fat cheese Dinner: 60g of baked salmon 2 tablespoons of cooked mixed vegetables (courgettes, carrots) Considerations: Fluid intake: Drink at least 1.5 liters of water a day, avoiding drinking during meals to avoid premature filling of the stomach. Supplements: It is essential to take the vitamin and mineral supplements prescribed by your doctor to avoid nutritional deficiencies. Portions: Portions must be very small; Always consult your doctor or nutritionist to customize quantities based on your specific needs.

FUTURE AND CONCLUSION OF THE BARIATRIC DIET

Future of Bariatric Surgery Bariatric surgery has already revolutionized the treatment of severe obesity and associated conditions, but the future of this discipline promises further significant advances. These advances are driven by new technologies, innovative research and an ever-increasing focus on personalizing care. 1. Technological Innovations Minimally Invasive Surgery: Laparoscopic and robotic techniques will continue to evolve, making surgeries even less invasive, reducing recovery times and minimizing associated risks. Telemedicine and Remote Monitoring: Postoperative monitoring could increasingly be managed through telemedicine, allowing patients to receive remote support and monitoring, reducing the need for in-person visits. 2. Personalization of Care Tailored Treatments:

With the advancement of precision medicine, it will be possible to personalize surgical and nutritional protocols based on the patient's genetic and metabolic characteristics, optimizing results. Psychology and Behavioral Support: The integration of psychological support and tailored behavioral change programs will be key to helping patients manage long-term nutrition and lifestyle challenges post-surgery. 3. New Approaches and Techniques Non-Surgical Techniques: New, less invasive treatments, such as advanced intragastric balloons or endoscopic devices, may emerge, offering alternatives to surgery for some patients. Microbiome and Metabolism Research: Research on the gut microbiome and its role in metabolism could lead to new treatments combined with bariatric surgery to improve weight management and metabolic health. 4. Accessibility and Inclusion Broadening

Access: Access to bariatric surgery is expected to expand, especially in developing countries, thanks to education and funding programs that make treatments more accessible. Reduced Stigma: With increased awareness and acceptance of obesity as a complex medical condition, the stigma associated with bariatric surgery may reduce, encouraging more people to consider this treatment option. Conclusion Bariatric surgery represents a powerful ally in the fight against severe obesity and associated metabolic diseases, offering millions of people a new chance to live a healthier and more active life. However, long-term success depends not only on the surgery, but also on the patient's commitment to following an appropriate eating plan and lifestyle. Perseverance and Support:

The post-surgical road is an ongoing journey that requires perseverance, patience and support. It is essential that patients work closely with a multidisciplinary team, including doctors, nutritionists, psychologists and exercise specialists, to address challenges and ensure lasting success. Continuous Evolution: With the evolution of technology and medicine, bariatric surgery will continue to improve, offering increasingly effective and less invasive solutions. This discipline does not just represent a surgical solution, but a real life change, which, if approached with the right spirit and support, can lead to extraordinary results. In summary, the future of bariatric surgery is promising and full of possibilities. With the adoption of new technologies and a personalized approach, patients will be able to benefit from increasingly better results, contributing to a greater quality of life and lasting general well-being.

BREAKFAST RECIPES

31

EGG WHITE OMELETTE WITH SPINACH AND RICOTTA

Preparation time: 10 minutes

Cooking time: 15-20 minutes

Doses: 4 people

Ingredients:

8 egg whites

200g of fresh spinach

100g of ricotta

50g of grated Parmigiano Reggiano

1 clove of garlic

Salt, pepper and nutmeg to taste

1 tablespoon extra virgin olive oil

Preparation

Wash the spinach, chop it coarsely and cook it in a pan with a drizzle of oil and the chopped garlic until it softens. In a bowl, beat the egg whites with a fork, add the ricotta, parmesan, salt, pepper and nutmeg. Add the spinach to the egg mixture and mix well. Pour the mixture into a non-stick pan greased with oil and cook over medium heat, covering with a lid. When the omelette is set on the bottom, turn it over with the help of a plate or a spatula. Cook the other side until golden brown.

BERRY PROTEIN SMOOTHIE

Preparation time: 5 minutes

Cooking time: Not necessary

Doses: 1 person

Ingredients:

150g of Greek yogurt

1 scoop protein powder (flavor of your choice)

100g of mixed berries (fresh or frozen)

1/2 banana

150ml vegetable milk (almond, soy, rice)

Natural sweetener to taste (stevia, erythritol)

Preparation

Place all the ingredients in a blender and blend until smooth. If you prefer it sweeter, add sweetener. Tips: For a lighter version, you can reduce the amount of ricotta or protein powder. If you are lactose intolerant, use vegetable milk and soy yogurt.

BANANA PROTEIN PANCAKES

Preparation time: 10 minutes

Cooking time: About 2 minutes per pancake

Servings: 4 people (about 8 pancakes)

Ingredients:

2 ripe bananas

4 egg whites

100g of oatmeal

1 teaspoon baking powder

Cinnamon powder to taste

Coconut oil or non-stick spray

to grease the pan

Preparation

Mash the bananas with a fork until you get a puree. In a bowl, combine the mashed banana, egg whites, oat flour, baking powder and cinnamon. Mix well until you obtain a homogeneous mixture. Heat a nonstick pan and lightly grease it with coconut oil or spray. Pour a ladle of mixture for each pancake and cook over medium heat until bubbles form on the surface and the edge is golden. Flip the pancake and cook the other side. Repeat the operation until the mixture is finished.

GREEK YOGURT WITH PUREE OF APPLE AND CINNAMON

Preparation time: 5 minutes

Cooking time: Not necessary

Doses: 4 people

Ingredients:

500g of Greek yogurt

2 apples

1 teaspoon ground cinnamon

Chopped hazelnuts (optional)

Preparation

Peel the apples, cut them into pieces and cook them in a pan with a little water until they are soft. Mash the apples with a fork to obtain a puree. Pour the Greek yogurt into four bowls. Add a spoonful of applesauce and a sprinkle of cinnamon to each bowl. Decorate with chopped hazelnuts, if desired.

Tips: For apple puree, you can also use other types of fruit, such as pears or plums.

OAT PORRIDGE AND ALMOND MILK

Preparation time: 5 minutes

Cooking time: 2-3 minutes

Doses: 2 person

Ingredients:

80g of oat flakes

400ml of almond milk

Fresh fruit to taste (bananas, blueberries, strawberries)

Seeds (chia, flax, pumpkin)

Chopped walnuts or almonds

Ground cinnamon

Honey or agave syrup (optional)

Preparation

In a saucepan, pour the oat flakes and almond milk. Cook over low heat, stirring constantly, until the porridge has reached the desired consistency. Pour the porridge into a bowl and add the chopped fruit, seeds, nuts, cinnamon and sweeten with honey or agave syrup, if desired.

Advice:

You can customize your porridge with different fruits, seeds and nuts.

SCRAMBLED EGGS WITH AVOCADO AND CHERRY TOMATOES

Preparation time: 5 minutes

Cooking time: 5 minutes

Doses: 2 person

Ingredients:

4 eggs

1 ripe avocado

4 cherry tomatoes

Salt and pepper to taste

Extra virgin olive oil

Preparation

In a non-stick pan, heat a drizzle of oil. Beat the eggs in a bowl with a pinch of salt and pepper. Pour the eggs into the pan and cook them over low heat, stirring constantly with a fork, until you get soft scrambled eggs. In the meantime, cut the avocado into cubes and the cherry tomatoes in half. Add the avocado and cherry tomatoes to the scrambled eggs and mix gently.

Advice:

For scrambled eggs, you can add other vegetables like spinach or mushrooms.

CHIA PUDDING WITH COCONUT AND BLUEBERRIES

Preparation time: 5 minutes

Rest time: At least 2 hours

Servings: 2

Ingredients:

2 tablespoons of chia seeds

1 cup coconut milk

1/4 cup fresh or frozen blueberries

1 tablespoon honey (optional)

Grated zest of one lime (optional)

Preparation

Combine the ingredients: In a jar or bowl, add the chia seeds, coconut milk, blueberries, honey and lime zest (if using). Mix well: Mix all the ingredients well until the chia seeds are completely immersed in the liquid. Rest: Cover the jar and leave to rest in the refrigerator for at least 2 hours, or until the pudding has reached the desired consistency. Serve: Serve the chia pudding decorating with some fresh blueberries.

Advice:

Chia Pudding: You can customize your pudding by adding other berries, nuts or seeds.

MINI ZUCCHINI AND CHEESE FRITTERS

Preparation time: 20 minutes

Cooking time: 15 minutes

Servings: About 12 pancakes

Ingredients:

1 grated courgette

100g of grated cheese

(like grana padano)

1 egg

50g of 00 flour

1 teaspoon baking powder

Salt and pepper to taste

Frying oil

Preparation

Prepare the dough: In a bowl, combine the grated courgette, grated cheese, egg, flour, yeast, salt and pepper. Mix well until you obtain a homogeneous mixture. Form the pancakes: With the help of two teaspoons, form small balls of dough. Fry: Heat plenty of oil in a pan and fry the pancakes until they are golden on both sides. Drain the pancakes on absorbent paper to remove excess oil.

Advice:

Mini Fritters: You can add other vegetables to the dough, such as carrots or spinach.

TOFU AND MIXED VEGETABLES OMELETTE

Preparation time: 15 minutes

Cooking time: 10 minutes

Servings: 2

Ingredients:

200g of tofu

1 onion

1 pepper

1 courgette

1 egg

2 tablespoons chickpea flour

1 tablespoon soy milk

**Salt, pepper, aromatic herbs
to taste (oregano, basil)**

Extra virgin olive oil

Preparation

Prepare the vegetables: Finely slice the onion, pepper and courgette. Crumble the tofu: Crumble the tofu with a fork. Combine the ingredients: In a bowl, combine the crumbled tofu, egg, chickpea flour, soy milk, vegetables, salt, pepper and herbs. Mix well until you obtain a homogeneous mixture. Cook the omelette: Heat a non-stick pan with a drizzle of oil. Pour the mixture and cook over medium heat, covering with a lid, until golden brown underneath. Flip the omelette and cook the other side too.

COTTAGE CHEESE WITH STRAWBERRIES AND LIGHT HONEY

Preparation time: 5 minutes

Cooking time: Not necessary

Servings: 1

Ingredients:

100g of cottage cheese

150g of strawberries

1 tablespoon light honey

Fresh mint (optional)

Preparation

Wash and cut the fruit: Wash the strawberries and cut them in half. Assemble the dish: Place the cottage cheese in a bowl, add the cut strawberries and season with light honey. Decorate: Complete the dish with a few fresh mint leaves.

Advice:

Cottage cheese: You can replace the cottage cheese with Greek yogurt or ricotta for a higher protein option.

RECIPES APPETIZERS AND SMOOTHIES

CHICKEN AND AVOCADO SALAD

Preparation time: 15 minutes

Servings: 1

Ingredients:

100g of grilled chicken breast

and cut into cubes

1/2 ripe avocado, cut into cubes

1/4 cucumber, cut into rounds

1/4 red onion, finely sliced

1 cherry tomato, cut into cubes

2 tablespoons of corn

1 tablespoon sunflower seeds

2 tablespoons vinaigrette

(or lemon, oil and salt

Preparation

In a bowl, combine all the ingredients.

Seasoned with vinaigrette or with an emulsion of lemon, oil and salt.

Stir gently to blend the flavors.

Advice:

Salad: You can customize the salad by adding other ingredients such as arugula, spinach, walnuts or feta cheese.

BLENDED VEGETABLE SOUP

Preparation time: 20 minutes

Cooking time: 20 minutes

Servings: 2

Ingredients:

1 carrot

1 potato

1/2 onion

1 stick of celery

1 liter of vegetable broth

Extra virgin olive oil

Salt and pepper to taste

Fresh aromatic herbs

(parsley, basil)

Preparation

Wash and cut the vegetables into pieces. In a pan, heat a drizzle of oil and fry the onion. Add the other vegetables and cook for a few minutes. Pour in the vegetable broth, salt, pepper and cook until the vegetables are tender. Blend everything with an immersion blender until you obtain a smooth cream. Serve the soup hot, decorating with a drizzle of oil and a few leaves of aromatic herbs.

Tips: Soup: For a creamier soup, you can add a spoonful of Greek yogurt or ricotta. You can also vary the vegetables according to the season.

BANANA SMOOTHIE

Difficulty: Very easy

Preparation: 10 min

Serves: 4 people

Cost: very low

ingredients

Bananas 300 g

Ice 60 g

cinnamon sticks 2 g

Whole milk 150 g

Preparation

To make the banana milkshake, peel the bananas and cut them into small pieces, then place the freshly cut banana pieces into the blender. Add cinnamon, ice cubes and cold milk. Operate the mixer until you obtain a thick and creamy mixture. Pour the mixture into glasses and garnish with cinnamon sticks. Serve the banana smoothie immediately and enjoy it cold!

CUCUMBER SMOOTHIE AND LIME AND TURMERIC YOGURT

Time 10 min

ingredients

2 people

300 g of low-fat yogurt

260 g of Greek yogurt

200 g of peeled cucumber

30 g of fresh ginger

1 lime

turmeric

cucumber slices

salt

Preparation

For the cucumber, lime and turmeric smoothie recipe, blend together the low-fat yogurt, 200 g of Greek yogurt, the peeled cucumber, the sliced ginger, 1 teaspoon of turmeric, the juice and the grated zest of the lime. Divide the remaining yogurt between 2 tall glasses, then fill with the smoothie. Top with cucumber slices.

ORANGES, SWORDFISH AND SPINACH WITH MUSTARD

Time 25 min

ingredients

for 4 people

300 g of sliced smoked swordfish

3 oranges

fresh spinach

mint

mustard

vinegar

pink pepper

extra virgin olive oil

Preparation

For the recipe of oranges, swordfish and spinach with mustard, peel the oranges (remove the peel following the contour of the fruit with a small knife, so as to remove the white peel). Then cut them into slices about 5 mm thick. Arrange them on a tray together with the slices of smoked swordfish, spinach leaves and a few mint leaves. Mix 1 teaspoon of mustard with 4 tablespoons of oil and 1 tablespoon of vinegar. Season the salad with this mixture and finish with pink peppercorns.

PUNTARELLE AND FRIED ANCHOVIES SALAD

Time 40 min

ingredients

for 4 people

300 g of chicory

18 fresh anchovies

re-milled durum wheat semolina

lemon

Peanut oil

extra virgin olive oil

salt

pepper

Preparation

For the chicory and fried anchovy salad recipe, prepare the chicory. Puntarelle is located in the heart of the Catalan capital. To clean them, remove the outer leaves (which you can use in soups or omelettes). Remove the ribs from the head, remove the base and cut them into thin strips, then place them in water and ice for 1520 minutes. Clean the anchovies: remove the head, open them like a book, remove the bones, gut them, rinse and dry them with kitchen paper. Then flour them in the semolina and fry them quickly in a pan with hot peanut oil. Drain them on kitchen paper and add salt. Drain the chicory, dry them and season them with the juice of 1/2 lemon, 45 tablespoons of extra virgin olive oil, salt and pepper. Serve Enjoy your meal.

CARROT HUMMUS WITH YOGURT AND SPICY OIL

Time 1h

ingredients

6 people servings

500 g of carrots

200 g of cherry tomatoes

120 g of boiled cannellini beans

80 g of Greek yogurt

1 fresh chili pepper

1 lemon, garlic

sweet paprika

extra virgin olive oil

salt and pepper

Preparation

Peel the carrots, cut them into slices and boil them in boiling salted water for 40 minutes; drain them and keep the cooking water aside. Cut the cherry tomatoes in half lengthwise, place them on a grill and bake at 180°C for 15 minutes; remove from the oven and season with a drizzle of oil, a pinch of salt and freshly ground pepper. Blend the cannellini beans with the juice of 1/2 lemon, the carrots and a ladle of their cooking liquid. Using an immersion blender, blend 60 g of oil with the chilli pepper removed from the seeds and cut into slices, 1/4 of a clove of garlic and 1 teaspoon of sweet paprika. Distribute the carrot hummus on plates, stain it with yogurt and drops of chilli oil, and serve with cherry tomatoes and, if desired, with croutons, breadsticks or crispy vegetable sticks.

BUTTER WITH SAUCE

AND BEET CHIPS

Time 25 min

ingredients

for 8 people

250 g of already boiled beets

250 g of soft salted butter

25 g of desalted capers

8 pickled gherkins

beetroot chips and

carrot (on sale ready-made)

vinegar, mustard, chives

chervil, mini baguette

white bread

extra virgin olive oil

sugar, salt, pepper

Preparation

For the butter with sauce and beetroot chips recipe, cut the beetroot into slices, already boiled and blended finely with 15 g of vinegar, 20 g of oil, a pinch of salt and a pinch of sugar, pepper, a slice of bread without the rind, 3 gherkins, 15 g of capers and 1 teaspoon of mustard. Divide the soft butter into small pieces, collect it in a bowl and work it with a spoon until it takes on a soft and creamy consistency. Distribute it on a cutting board, spread it with a spatula with soft movements, and complete with the beetroot sauce, 45 gherkins cut in half lengthwise, 1 tablespoon of capers, carrot and beetroot chips, chives cut into wedges, and a a few chervil leaves. Serve with mini baguettes.

FRUIT SMOOTHIE

Preparation: 10 min

Serves: 2 people

Low cost

ingredients

2 peaches

2 bananas

200 g of strawberries

2 kiwis

60 ml of whole milk

Preparation

To prepare the fruit smoothie, start by peeling the kiwi, then cut it into cubes, eliminating the central white part. Wash the peaches, peel them and cut them into cubes. Wash the strawberries, remove the green stem and cut them in half, finally peel the bananas and cut them into slices. Place all the fruit in the glass of a blender and add the milk. Blend until you obtain a smooth and homogeneous mixture. Serve now!

CHICKEN MEATBALLS WITH TURMERIC

Time 40 min

ingredients

for 4 people

300 g clean

chicken breast

1 lemon, 1 egg

1 egg white

turmeric powder

panko bread

fresh cream

Peanut oil

salt and pepper

Preparation

For the turmeric chicken meatballs recipe, cut the chicken into small pieces and blend it with a pinch of salt, 1 egg, 3 tablespoons of cream, 1 tablespoon of turmeric powder, 1 tablespoon of lemon juice and the zest of 1/2 2 lemon. Form the proceeds into about 30 meatballs the size of olives. Dip them in the beaten egg white, then in the panko, and fry them in very hot oil (180°C) for 2 minutes, a few at a time. Drain them on kitchen paper and serve.

PRAWNS WITH HONEY AND BREAD SPICESBREAD

Time 30 min

+ 40min marinade

ingredients

for 4 people

250 g of cleaned prawn tails

50 g 3 slices of gingerbread

1 medium shallot

1 lime, fresh ginger

fresh chili pepper

white sesame seeds

dry white wine

Honey

extra virgin olive oil

mixed salad, salt

Preparation

Prepare the marinade: grate 50 g of fresh ginger into a fairly large bowl. Add 2 tablespoons of honey, 10 g of sesame seeds, the shallot cut into thin slices, 1 chopped and seeded chilli pepper, a pinch of salt, the juice of 1/2 lime and 30 g of dry white wine. Mix the prawn tails well with the marinade to evenly flavor; cover the bowl with cling film and leave to rest for 40 minutes at room temperature. Blend or crumble the gingerbread (if you prefer less sweet flavors you can use another bread;

an excellent alternative is rye bread, which will counteract the spicy sweet-acid flavor of the marinade). Toast the crumbs in a hot, dry pan over medium-low heat, or in the oven on a baking tray covered with baking paper at 150°C for 15 minutes. Once cold it will be crunchy. Lastly, sauté the prawns in the same hot pan with all the marinade for 23 minutes. Serve hot or warm sprinkled with crunchy gingerbread crumbs and complete with a mixed salad dressed with a drizzle of oil and salt.

FENNEL CREAM
WITH GINGER E
FRIED ARTICHOKES

Time 40 min

ingredients

for 4 people

500 g of peeled fennel

500 g of vegetable broth

10 g of fresh ginger

3 slices of homemade bread

2 artichokes

1 large potato

1 bay leaf, mixed seeds

Rice flour

extra virgin olive oil

seed oil, salt

Preparation

For the recipe for fennel soup with ginger and fried artichokes, peel the potato and cut it into chunks. Cut the fennel into thin wedges. Peel the ginger, grate it and squeeze the pulp to obtain the juice. Heat a drizzle of oil in a pan, flavor with bay leaves and brown the potato and fennel for 1 minute; add the vegetable broth and ginger juice, add salt and continue cooking for another 20 minutes. Finally, remove the bay leaf and blend everything. Clean the artichokes and cut the hearts into thin strips;

Flour them and fry them in plenty of hot seed oil for about 4 minutes, then drain them on kitchen paper. Cut the slices of bread into cubes, remove the crust, grease them with a drizzle of oil and brown in the oven at 170°C for about 4 minutes. Distribute the fennel cream onto the plates and complete with the mixed seeds, crunchy artichokes and browned bread cubes. Season to taste with freshly ground pepper and serve.

AZUKI BEAN HUMMUS

Preparation: 5 min

Doses for: 4 people

ingredients

250g cooked adzuki beans

1 tablespoon tahini

1 tablespoon apple cider vinegar

½ teaspoon oregano

1 pinch of garlic

1 pinch of salt

Preparation

Pour the adzuki beans, tahini, apple cider vinegar, oregano, garlic and salt into the food processor and start blending, adding half a glass of water if the mixture is too dry. Blend everything until you obtain a perfectly smooth cream. Our azuki bean hummus is ready to be enjoyed accompanied by a slice of bread, a polenta crouton or your favorite raw vegetables, such as carrots, celery and fennel.

CARROT AND LIME SMOOTHIE

Doses for: 4 People

5 minutes of preparation

ingredients

Carrots 4

files 1

Mint 3 leaves

Brown sugar 1 handful

Preparation

Cut the carrots into rather small pieces, to put in a blender. Add the whole lime without the peel and the mint leaves, then a handful of brown sugar Carrot and lime smoothie, Turn on the blender and blend until you obtain a light orange juice.

SUPER ENERGY SMOOTHIE

Doses for: 4 People

5 minutes of preparation

ingredients

Parsley 1 sprig

Golden Delicious apples 1

Carrots 3

Cabbage 3 leaves

Preparation

Carrots, Cut the carrots into fairly small pieces and place them in a rather large container. Diced apple, Add the chopped cabbage leaves and the apple cut into pieces. Then transfer everything into the blender, turn on the mixer, and blend until you obtain a mixture. rather thick mixture, to be served immediately on the table.

MELON AND PEACH SMOOTHIE

Difficulty: Easy

Doses for: 4 People

5 minutes of preparation

ingredients

Melon 1 slice

Yellow peaches 1

Lemons 2

spoons Apricots 1

Carrots 3

Preparation

Cut the carrots into rather small pieces and place them in a bowl together with the pieces of melon. Cut the apricot and peach into pieces and add them to the container with two tablespoons of lemon juice, blend the melon, peach, then transfer everything into a blender. and blend until you obtain a fragrant and colored juice, serve.

BLACK CABBAGE CHIPS WITH SESAME AND GOAT SEEDS

Time 15 min

ingredients

for 4 people

300 g of black cabbage

250 g of goat's cheese

1 organic lemon

toasted sesame seeds

extra virgin olive oil

pink pepper, salt

Preparation

For the kale chips with sesame seeds and goat cheese, peel the kale leaves, pat dry and dry. Season them with a drizzle of oil and salt and place them in the microwave in frying mode for 1 minute and 30 seconds. Or place them between two sheets of microwave baking paper and cook at 600 W for 1 minute and then at maximum power for another 30 seconds, checking when they are crispy. Sprinkle with sesame. Mix the goat cheese with a drizzle of oil and the grated lemon zest. Serve the chips sprinkled with sesame seeds, sprigs of goat's cheese and a little coarsely ground pink pepper. Be careful, each microwave oven has different powers. The cooking minutes must therefore be calculated based on the power of your appliance.

SAUTE RICE CAKES WITH MUSHROOMS

Time 90 min

ingredients

for 8 people

300 grams of rice

300 g pumpkin pulp

150 g of taleggio cheese

160 g of cleaned porcini mushrooms

100 g of clean pleurotus mushrooms

80 g of cleaned chanterelles

60 g parmesan

butter, garlic

lemon thyme

extra virgin olive oil

salt and pepper

Preparation

For the recipe for sautéed rice cakes with mushrooms, steam the pumpkin pulp in pieces for about 20 minutes. Blend into cream, adding salt at the end. Toast the rice in a fat-free saucepan, pour boiling water over it and cook like a risotto. 5 minutes after the end of cooking, add salt, add the pumpkin cream, complete cooking, remove from the heat and stir in the grated parmesan, a knob of butter and ground pepper. Roll out the still hot rice on a sheet of baking paper to a thickness of at least 1 cm, leveling it well, cut out 1416 discs of 10 cm in diameter (crackers), and let them cool completely;

You can also prepare them the day before.
Brown the biscuits (no more than 3 at a time)
with a knob of butter and 4 tablespoons of oil
in a pan, making them brown well on both
sides. Cut all the mushrooms into small
pieces and brown them in a pan covered in
oil and with 1 clove of garlic in its peel,
slightly crushed, for 45 minutes over high
heat. Immediately distribute the mushrooms
on the biscuits, complete with pieces of
taleggio (the heat of the mushrooms will
make it melt), lemon thyme and serve.

CAULIFLOWER MEATBALLS

Time 9/5 min

ingredients

Portions for 4 people

600 g of cleaned cauliflower

250 grams of potatoes

70 g parmesan

3 eggs

bread crumbs

Peanut oil

thyme, salt, pepper

Preparation

For the cauliflower meatballs recipe, boil the potatoes in their skins, then peel them and mash them in the potato masher while they are still hot. Cook the cauliflower florets in boiling water for 1520 minutes, so that they remain slightly crunchy. Leave to cool on kitchen paper. Chop the florets with the leaves of 2 sprigs of thyme in a blender and add them to the mashed potatoes. Also add 1 lightly beaten egg, the grated parmesan, salt and pepper. Mix everything until you obtain a homogeneous mixture. Form meatballs by working the mixture with your hands: if it is too soft you can add a little stale breadcrumbs. Dip in the other 2 beaten eggs, then in the breadcrumbs. Fry them in boiling oil until golden. Alternatively, place them on a baking tray covered with baking paper and cook at 175°C for about 15 minutes.

SEAFOOD PIE WITH ARTICHOKES

Time 90 min

ingredients

for 4 people

460 g 2 discs of

rolled out puff pastry

500 g clams

500 g of mussels

12 red prawns

6 artichokes

1 egg, lemon

white wine

extra virgin olive oil

parsley, garlic, salt

Preparation

Open the 2 puff pastry discs. Place the first
one, with its paper, on the oven tray. Form a
shell using rolled sheets of baking paper and
place the second sheet of shortcrust pastry
on top. Attach it along the edges to the first
disc and cut out a central opening, to create a
sort of rounded volcano. From the scraps,
make puff pastry balls and decorate the edge
of the hole. Brush everything with the beaten
egg and bake at 180°C for about 30 minutes.
Remove from the oven and gently remove
the baking paper from inside. Put the dome
back in the oven for 23 minutes if the inside
is still a little moist. Baked. Clean the
artichokes and cut them into segments,
gradually immersing them in water and
lemon. Drain them and cook them in a pan

with a drizzle of oil, 1 clove of garlic, a splash of white wine and salt, for about 15/20 minutes, adding a little water if necessary. Open the clams and mussels separately in two saucepans with a drizzle of oil, garlic and parsley: cover with the lid and cook until the shells open. Turn off and shell, keeping only a few whole molluscs to serve. Shell the prawns and clean them from the casing. Fry them in a pan with a drizzle of oil together with the heads, which will give more flavour, for 2 minutes. Remove the heads and add the shelled clams, mussels and artichokes to the pan. Mix everything. Fill the puff pastry shell with this filling, completing the upper part with the clams and mussels that you have kept in the shell.

RECIPES
FIRST DISHES

PUMPKIN AND ONION PUREE

Preparation time: 15 minutes

Cooking time: 30 minutes

Servings: 4

Ingredients:

1 kg of pumpkin

2 onions

50g of butter

200ml of milk

Salt, pepper, nutmeg to taste

Preparation

Prepare the vegetables: Peel the pumpkin and cut it into cubes. Finely slice the onions. Cook the vegetables: In a pan, sauté the onions in the butter. Add the squash and cook for about 20 minutes, or until tender. Blend everything: Blend the pumpkin and onions with an immersion blender or with a mixer until you obtain a smooth cream. Add the milk: Pour in the hot milk and blend again. Season with salt, pepper and nutmeg. Serve: Serve the mashed potatoes hot, decorating with a drizzle of oil and a sprinkling of parmesan (optional).

QUINOA RISOTTO WITH SPINACH

Preparation time: 10 minutes

Cooking time: 20 minutes

Servings: 4

Ingredients:

200g of quinoa

400ml of vegetable broth

400g of fresh spinach

1 clove of garlic

Extra virgin olive oil

Grated parmesan to taste

Salt, pepper to taste

Preparation

Toast the quinoa: In a pan, dry toast the quinoa for a few minutes, until it becomes slightly golden and releases its aroma. Cook the quinoa: Add the hot vegetable broth and cook over low heat for about 15 minutes, or until the quinoa is cooked and the liquid is absorbed. Prepare the spinach: In the meantime, wash and cut the spinach. In a pan, fry the garlic in a drizzle of oil and add the spinach. Cook for a few minutes, until wilted. Combine everything: Add the spinach to the quinoa risotto, mix well and season with salt and pepper. Serve: Serve the risotto hot, sprinkling with grated parmesan.

CAVATELLI WITH CHICKPEAS, TURNIP TOPS AND POTATOES

Preparation: 15 min

Cooking time: 35 min

Serves: 4 people

ingredients

500 g of fresh cavatelli

300 g of turnip greens

200 g of potatoes

120 g of cooked chickpeas

1 shallot

1 clove of garlic

1 teaspoon chopped rosemary

kilos

Preparation

First, cut the turnip greens into small pieces and wash them well. Peel the potatoes and cut them into cubes, then slice the shallot. In a large non-stick pan, brown the garlic clove, rosemary and a pinch of chilli pepper in a little oil, then add the shallot and potatoes and cook for a couple of minutes. Cook the vegetables. Pour the turnip tops into the pan, add a little salt and cook with the lid on for 20 minutes or until the vegetables are soft. Add the chickpeas to the vegetables and continue cooking for another 5 minutes. Season the cavatelli In the meantime, boil the cavatelli in plenty of lightly salted boiling water, drain them al dente and reserve a cup of the cooking water. Sauté the pasta together with the vegetables, adding a little pasta cooking water to mix everything well,

PAPPARDELLE WITH RADICCHIO SAUCE, FIGS

Preparation: 10 min

Cooking: 20 min

Serves: 4 people

ingredients

350 g of pappardelle

1 large head of radicchio

67 large, ripe figs

10 sage leaves

3 bay leaves

Preparation

Chop the sage very finely. Separately, cut the radicchio into strips, peel the figs and cut them into cubes. In a large pan, heat a add a drizzle of extra virgin olive oil together with the chopped sage and bay leaves and brown for 12 minutes on a low heat. fry for 5 minutes over medium-high heat until golden brown. At this point add the radicchio and figs and continue cooking for another 5 minutes, adding salt to taste. Skip the pasta. Boil the pappardelle in abundant salted water, drain them al dente, and sauté them in the pan with the sauce for 12 minutes so that they gain flavour, adding, if necessary, a drop of the pasta cooking water. Turn off the heat and serve immediately while the pasta is hot.

WHOLE WHOLE FUSILLI WITH EDAMAME PESTO E SUNFLOWER SEEDS

Preparation: 10 min

Cooking: 20 min

Serves: 4 people

ingredients

360 g of wholemeal fusilli

200 g of edamame

40 g of sunflower seeds

70 g of rocket

1 tablespoon basil pesto

2 tablespoons lemon juice

60 g of black olives, salt and pepper

Extra virgin olive oil

Preparation

Start by blanching the edamame in lightly salted boiling water for about ten minutes or until they soften. Drain them and run under cold water to prevent them from cooking. Boil the pasta. Boil the wholemeal fusilli in plenty of lightly salted water and drain them al dente, keeping a cup of the cooking water. Prepare the pesto In a food processor, blend the rocket with a drizzle of oil and a few tablespoons of the pasta cooking water until a perfectly smooth mixture is obtained, then add the edamame, sunflower seeds, basil pesto, lemon juice and a good drizzle of oil, season with salt and pepper and blend everything until a pesto is formed that is not perfectly smooth but rather soft, diluting it if necessary with a little pasta cooking water. Season the fusilli with the edamame and sunflower seed pesto,

PENNE COURGETTE SPECK AND CHEESE

Easy difficulty

Average cost

Preparation time 10 minutes

Cooking time 10 minutes

2 servings

ingredients

200 g penne

5 courgettes

1 clove of garlic

taste the pepper

taste the salt

to taste the oil

extra virgin olive oil

100 g of spreadable cheese

50 g of almonds

100 g of grated cheese

speck 150 g

Preparation

Penne with courgettes, speck and cheese, to prepare this recipe we start with the courgettes, wash them carefully, then cut them in half and boil them for a few minutes. In the meantime, put a drizzle of oil and a clove of garlic in a pan. Fry, then remove and add the speck, leave to cook for a few minutes and add the wine. In the meantime, take the other courgettes and cut them into slices, add them to the speck, season with salt and pepper and cook over high heat.

We take the boiled courgettes, put them in the bowl, add the salt, pepper, spreadable cheese, extra virgin olive oil and almonds, and blend everything thus obtaining a smooth and homogeneous cream, which we leave aside. Let's cook the pasta. Once cooked, drain it, sauté it with the courgette speck, add the cream, the grated cheese and leave to macerate. We serve, and here are my super Penne with courgettes, speck and cheese ready to be enjoyed.

PENS WITH PRIMBS
AND TOMATOES

Easy difficulty

Average cost

Preparation time 10 minutes

Cooking time 15 minutes

2 servings

ingredients

200 g penne

300 g of prawns

taste the salt

taste the pepper

try the extra virgin olive oil

300 g of cherry tomatoes

1/2 glass of white wine

2 tablespoons cream cheese

basil leaves

Preparation

Penne with prawns and cherry tomatoes, for this recipe we start by washing the cherry tomatoes, carefully cleaning the prawns, and removing the carapace and intestinal casing, which we find both on the belly and on the back. Take a pan, add a drizzle of oil and the chopped garlic clove, let it brown, then add the prawns, fry and add the wine. In the meantime, take the tomatoes,

Cut them into cubes and, once the wine has evaporated, add them to the fish with the basil leaves. Season with salt and pepper and leave to cook for about 10 minutes, then add the spreadable cheese and let it melt. We cook the pasta in plenty of salted water, serve it on a serving dish, and here are my Penne with prawns and tomatoes, ready to be enjoyed.

TAGLIATELLE WITH COURGETTES SPECK RICOTTA

Easy difficulty

Average cost

Preparation time 10 minutes

Cooking time 15 minutes

4 servings

ingredients

500 g of pasta tagliatelle

4 very fresh courgettes

150 g of diced speck

1 clove of garlic

1/2 glass of white wine

try the extra virgin olive oil

150 g of ricotta

to taste Salt to taste. pepper

For the batter

1 egg, to taste 00 flour

taste the cold water

to taste Salt to taste. pepper

Preparation

Tagliatelle with courgettes and speck ricotta, for this first course we start with the courgettes, wash them carefully, cut two into cubes, two into slices, and prepare the batter. We prepare the batter by eye, put the egg in a bowl, add salt and pepper and mix with a whisk. Add about 3 tablespoons of flour, mix and dilute with cold water. At this point we immerse the courgette slices, and when we have hot oil we fry them. When they are golden brown, place them on baking paper, adding a little salt. In a pan, put a drizzle of oil with a clove of garlic, let it brown, then remove it and add the speck, fry, add the wine, and when it has evaporated, add the courgettes, cook over high heat, season with salt and pepper. In the meantime, mix the ricotta with a drizzle of oil, salt, pepper and a little water, if cooked better, and set aside. Bring salted water to the boil, add the pasta and boil. We take our tagliatelle, sauté them with the courgettes, add the ricotta cream, and serve with the fried courgettes.

BROWN RICE WITH LEMON WALNUTS AND PARSLEY

Preparation: 10 min

Cooking: 15 min

Serves: 4 people

ingredients

320 g of brown rice

1 lemon

90 g of walnuts

3 tablespoons of parsley

fresh mince

1 pinch of pepper

1 pinch of saffron

Preparation

Boil the rice in plenty of salted water for 15 minutes or until cooked. In the meantime, toast the walnuts in a pan or in the oven at 180°C for 10 minutes until golden, chop coarsely with a knife, then add the parsley. Season the rice. Drain the rice and season it with a drizzle of oil, saffron, chilli pepper, walnuts, parsley and lemon juice and zest. Mix well to combine all the ingredients and serve hot or cold.

WHOLE WHOLE SPAGHETTI WITH AUBERGINES SAUCE

Preparation: 10 min

Cooking: 30 min

Serves: 4 people

ingredients

350 g of wholemeal spaghetti

400 g of aubergines

600 g of tomato pulp

1 tablespoon oregano

78 fresh basil leaves

1 clove of garlic

1 pinch of pepper

Preparation

First, heat a drizzle of oil in a large non-stick pan with the garlic, oregano and chilli.

pepper. When the oil is hot, add the aubergines, previously washed and cut into cubes, and brown them over medium-high heat for about ten minutes, together with a pinch of salt. We complete the sauce. When they are golden and slightly softened, add the tomato pulp and a drop of water, season with salt and cook for about twenty minutes with the lid on. Season the pasta In the meantime, boil the spaghetti and drain them al dente, keeping a glass of the pasta cooking water. Sauté in the aubergine sauce for a couple of minutes, adding a little cooking water if necessary if the sauce dries out too much. Finally, add the chopped basil and serve immediately, finishing with a sprinkling of grated cheese if desired.

POTATO GNOCCHI WITH PEPPER CREAM

Easy difficulty

Economical cost

Preparation time 10 minutes

Cooking time 5 minutes

2 servings

ingredients

500 g of fresh gnocchi

1 red pepper

1 yellow pepper

100 g of ricotta

150 g diced sweet bacon

taste the salt

taste the pepper

1/2 glass of white wine

100 g of grated cheese

Preparation

We take the peppers, wash them carefully, clean them and cut them coarsely. We take a pan, add a drizzle of oil and a clove of garlic, and let them cook for a few minutes. Once ready we can transfer them into the mixer glass, add salt, pepper, extra virgin olive oil, ricotta and cheese, and blend everything well, we will obtain a very soft cream, cover and set aside. In the same pan, add a drizzle of oil and a clove of garlic, and once browned, remove it and add the bacon, brown it then add the wine, and when it is crispy remove it from the heat, lay one part on absorbent paper. Cook the gnocchi, 2 minutes will be enough, drain them and sauté them in the bacon, add the pepper cream and leave to infuse, here are our gnocchi, ready to serve.

WINTER MINESTRONE WITH PASSATELLI BALLS

Time 50 minutes

ingredients

6 people servings

400 g of potatoes

250 g of Brussels sprouts

200 g of carrots

120 g grated parmesan

120 g of breadcrumbs

60 g of kale

60 g of colored beets

3 eggs, 1 leek, lemon, nutmeg

extra virgin olive oil

vegetable broth, salt

Preparation

Mix the eggs with the grated parmesan, breadcrumbs, a pinch of nutmeg, salt and grated lemon zest. Gather this dough into a loaf and let it rest for 1 hour wrapped in cling film, then shape into balls. Clean the leek and cut it into slices; peel the carrots and cut them into small pieces, clean the sprouts and cut them in half, peel the potatoes and cut them into cubes; cleaned and chopped, the cabbage and the chard. Wash all the vegetables. Brown the leek in a saucepan with a few tablespoons of oil for 2 minutes, then add the carrots and sprouts and, after 1 minute, the potatoes and 1.5 liters of broth. Cook for 2025 minutes, then add the watercress, cabbage and chard and cook for a further 10 minutes. Finally add the balls, boil them for 2 minutes and serve.

ARTICHOKE PARMIGIANA

Time 1h 10 min

ingredients

8 people

500 g of tomato puree

50 g grated parmesan

8 artichokes

2 eggs, lemon

1 golden onion

flour, basil

extra virgin olive oil

peanut oil, salt

Preparation

For the artichoke parmigiana recipe, clean the artichokes and cut them into slices about 3 mm thick; immerse yourself little by little in a basin of water acidulated with the juice of 1/2 lemon. Chop the onion and brown it in a pan with a drizzle of extra virgin olive oil; add the tomato puree and cook for 1015 minutes; flavor with a few basil leaves and a pinch of salt. the grated parmesan. Drain the artichokes, dry them, flour them and dip them in the beaten eggs; fry them in very hot peanut oil (170°C) for 34 minutes; dry the artichokes on kitchen paper and add a little salt. Arrange the ingredients in layers in a lasagna pan: first the tomato sauce, then the artichokes and 1 tablespoon of grated parmesan. Repeat the operation until the ingredients are used up. Bake at 180°C for 2025 minutes.

COLD PASTA WITH OLIVES, GRILLED AUBERGINES E ALMOND PESTO

Preparation: 15 min

Cooking: 15 min

Serves: 4 people

ingredients

320 g of short pasta

1 aubergine

90 g of olives

40 g of almonds

30 g of fresh basil

Extra virgin olive oil

Oregano, ½ clove of garlic

Preparation

Boil the pasta in plenty of salted water for the time indicated on the package, drain it and run it under cold water to cool it and stop cooking. Wash and slice the aubergines, then mix the extra virgin olive oil with the salt and oregano in a bowl. Brush the aubergines with the seasoning and grill for a few minutes on each side on a grill, then set them aside; once cold, cut them into fillets. Let's prepare the almond pesto. Cut the olives into slices, then toast the almonds for a few minutes in a non-stick pan, until they are lightly golden. At this point, blend the almonds with the basil, a drizzle of oil and the garlic until you obtain a completely smooth pesto. Season the pasta with the almond pesto, the sliced olives and the aubergines and, if desired, decorate each dish with some chopped almonds.

ORECCHIETTE WITH BROAD BEAN CREAM AND SAUTÉED CHICORY

Preparation: 20 min

Cooking: 20 min

Serves: 4 people

ingredients

320 g of orecchiette

400 g of freshly shelled broad beans

400 g of chicory

1 clove of garlic

1 pinch of pepper, ½ lemon

Preparation

First, clean the chicory well, cut it into large pieces and blanch for 5 minutes in lightly salted boiling water. Once cooked, drain the radicchio and sauté it in a pan with a clove of garlic and a pinch of chilli for a few minutes to flavor it. Let's prepare the broad bean cream. Boil the shelled broad beans for 5 minutes, drain them and transfer them to the tall glass of the immersion blender. Season with salt, pepper, a drizzle of oil and the juice of half a lemon and start blending with the immersion blender, adding just enough water to obtain a smooth and soft cream. Season the orecchiette. Boil the orecchiette in lightly salted boiling water, drain them al dente, keeping aside a glass of the cooking water, and toss them in the broad bean and chicory cream, adding a drop of cooking water if the sauce becomes too dry. Plate the orecchiette, complete each portion with a drizzle of raw oil and serve piping hot.

LEMON TAGLIOLINI WITH BASIL AND SAFFRON

Preparation: 5 min

Cooking time: 7 min

For 4 people

ingredients

500 g of fresh tagliolini

350 ml of cream of rice

2 lemons

1 and a half sachets of saffron

1 bunch of basil

Preparation

Prepare the sauce, boil plenty of salted water, add the tagliolini and cook them al dente. In the meantime, in a large pan, heat the rice cream with the saffron and a pinch of salt, then wash, dry and cut the basil into strips. Also wash and grate the zest of both lemons, and extract the juice only from one of the two. Pasta sauce Drain the pasta, reserving a glass of the cooking water. Dip the tagliatelle in the saffron cream and add the lemon zest and juice, the basil and a little cooking water until you obtain a smooth sauce. Serve immediately piping hot.

CANNELLINI BEAN SOUP

Preparation: 10 min

Cooking: 25 min

Serves: 4 people

ingredients

500 g of cannellini beans

already cooked beans

2 carrots, 1 onion

3 bay leaves

1 sprig of rosemary

200g unsweetened soy milk

1 pinch of pepper

1 clove of garlic

Vegetable broth

Preparation

Finely chop the onion, then wash the carrots, peel them with a potato peeler and cut them into rather small cubes. In a non-stick pan, fry the whole clove of garlic with a drizzle of oil, add the bay leaf and rosemary, and after about a minute also the onion and carrots, then season with a pinch of salt and fry for 10 minutes, until the vegetables are soft. We complete the soup, also add the beans and leave to flavor for 2 minutes, then add the soy milk and hot water or broth until everything is covered. Cook for 10 minutes, then season with a pinch of chilli and serve hot or warm.

RICE AND LENTIL SOUP

Preparation: 10 min

Cooking time: 45 min

Serves: 4 people

ingredients

200 g of brown rice

240 g of sautéed vegetables

(celery, carrots, onions)

130 g of lentils

3 bay leaves

a few sage leaves

2 sprigs of rosemary

2 tablespoons soy sauce

(gluten free if necessary)

1 piece of fresh ginger

vegetable broth

Preparation

In a large pan, heat a base of oil with the bay leaves, sage and chopped rosemary. Add the diced vegetables and cook for a few minutes. Add the brown rice and lentils, both previously rinsed under running water, cover with plenty of hot vegetable broth, bring to the boil and cook for approximately 4045 minutes. We complete the soup. Once both the lentils and rice are cooked, add salt and season with soy sauce and two tablespoons of ginger juice (which you can obtain by grating a small piece of fresh ginger and squeezing the pulp with your hands). At this point your soup is ready to be served piping hot.

COCONUT RICE WITH CHICKPEA CURRY

Time 40 min

ingredients

4 people

600 g of coconut milk

450 g of boiled chickpeas

200 g jasmine rice

40g grated coconut

2 cinnamon sticks

1 white onion, lime

fresh chili pepper

chilli flakes

curry, parsley

extra virgin olive oil

salt fine and coarse

Preparation

For the coconut rice with chickpea curry recipe, bring 300 g of water to the boil with 200 g of coconut milk and ½ teaspoon of coarse salt (be careful: when the coconut milk boils it swells a lot). Add the rice and cook it according to the times indicated on the package (1213 minutes) with the pan covered, without ever uncovering it. Slice the onion and fry it in a saucepan with a couple of tablespoons of oil, the cinnamon sticks (crush them lightly without breaking them), 45 slices of fresh chilli pepper and a pinch of salt for a couple of minutes, until it is slightly wilted. Add the chickpeas,

leave to flavor for 1 minute, then add the
first 2 teaspoons of curry and, after 1 minute,
400 g of coconut milk; continue cooking for
20 minutes, over low heat. Rehydrate the
grated coconut in 200 g of water for a few
minutes; squeeze it well and season it with
lime juice, a pinch of salt and a pinch of chilli
flakes; knead the mixture with your hands,
pinching a little with your fingers. Distribute
the rice on plates, season with the chickpea
curry, complete with the grated coconut,
chopped parsley and serve.

FENNEL AND CAVAGE SOUP WITH SPECK

Time 50 min

ingredients

4 people

460 g of cleaned fennel

400 g of cleaned cabbage

200 g of potatoes, 1 leek

60 g of homemade wholemeal bread

40 g of speck, 40 g of butter

extra virgin olive oil

salt and pepper

Preparation

For the recipe for fennel and cabbage soup with speck, set aside a few cabbage leaves, choosing the most tender one, and a few slices

of leek; chop the rest of the leek. Chop all the rest of the vegetables and collect them in a bowl. Brown the chopped leek in a saucepan with a drizzle of oil for 2 minutes; add the chopped vegetables, cook them, then add 1 liter of water and a pinch of salt. Cook for about 25 minutes over medium-low heat, then blend the soup and stir in the butter, adding salt and pepper. Brown the cabbage leaves and leek slices set aside in a pan with a drizzle of oil, browning them for a couple of minutes. Cut the bread into cubes and toast it in a pan with a knob of butter for a couple of minutes. Serve the soup with the toasted bread cubes and the sautéed vegetables, completing with the speck cut into strips.

PAVESE SOUP

Time 25 min

ingredients

4 people

500g chicken broth

400 g of stale bread

300 g grated parmesan

8 eggs

Marjoram

wise

thyme

salt

Preparation

For the Pavese soup recipe, bring the broth to the boil, add the chopped bread, the parmesan, 4 whole eggs and the finely chopped aromatic herbs; mix everything together with a hand whisk. Season with salt. Distribute the soup onto plates and complete each with 1 egg yolk, aromatic herb leaves, parmesan and, to taste, freshly ground pepper.

PASTA, BEANS, AND MUSSELS

Time 60 minutes

ingredients

4 people

1 kg of mussels

400 g of boiled cannellini beans

320 g mixed short pasta

2 cloves of garlic

1 bunch of fresh parsley

tomato paste

extra virgin olive oil

salt and pepper

Preparation

For the pasta, beans and mussels recipe, fry 1 clove of garlic in a pan with a couple of tablespoons of oil; add 1 teaspoon of tomato paste, leave to infuse, then add the beans with their cooking water, add salt and cook for about 40 minutes. Blend half the beans. Fry 1 clove of garlic in a saucepan with 2 tablespoons of oil; add the mussels and a few stalks of parsley; close with a lid and let the shells open. Shell the mussels, keeping some in their shells aside; filter their cooking water and add it to the blended beans, add 1 glass of water and cook the pasta according to the times indicated on the package, adding salt and pepper. Add the mussels and whole beans, then distribute them on the plates, complete with the chopped parsley, the mussels in their shells and a drizzle of oil.

CARDINAL'S TIMBALLO

Time 1h 30min

ingredients

10 people

2.5 kg of round tomatoes

800 g of tomato sauce

700 grams of mozzarella

500 g rigatoni

300 g of breadcrumbs

250 g grated parmesan

basil, oregano

parsley

extra virgin olive oil

salt and pepper

Preparation

For the Cardinal timbale recipe, cut the tomatoes horizontally, remove the seeds and place them on a baking tray covered with baking paper. Blend the breadcrumbs, basil, plenty of oregano and parsley, a glass of oil, salt and pepper. Heat the oven to 180°C. Stuff half the tomatoes with the mixture, and cook them in the oven until they are dry, even slightly burnt. Let cool. In the meantime, mix the grated parmesan with the diced mozzarella. Slowly thicken the tomato sauce flavored with salt, pepper and basil. Line a baking tray approximately 30cm in diameter with baking paper and grease it well.

Start arranging the tomatoes in a radial pattern starting from the center with the skin facing downwards. Position yourself, like a frame, also on the edges, compressing them so that they do not detach. Cook the rigatoni for 3 minutes in boiling water, drain them, pour them into the pan with the boiling tomato sauce, mix, cook them for another 3 minutes, add the parmesan and mozzarella and pour everything over the tomatoes in the pan, squeezing with your hands to don't stay empty. Place in the oven at 180°C for 45 minutes. Remove from the oven and let rest for about ten minutes. Turn out the timbale onto a serving plate. It is also delicious cold.

REGINETTE IN MONTEBORE WITH THREE PEPPER SAUCE

Time 35 min

ingredients

4 people

500 g of milk

350 g of long Reginette type pasta

100 g of Montebore cheese

flour, butter

black, pink and green peppercorns

salt

Preparation

For the recipe for queens in three-pepper Montebore sauce, coarsely grind 1 teaspoon of each grain of pepper (you can do it in the mortar or with a rolling pin, between two sheets of baking paper). Remove the crust from the montebore and cut it into small pieces. Melt 35 g of butter in a saucepan, mixing it with 35 g of flour; add a pinch of salt and the milk, slowly; Once the boil has risen, cook the béchamel for 34 minutes, stirring continuously. When it starts to "pull", add the montebore, stirring over low heat. Remove the sauce from the heat as soon as the cheese has melted. Boil the queens al dente, drain them and sauté them in the sauce, heat gently in a pan. Distribute the pasta onto plates, complete with the three peppers cut into pieces and serve immediately.

LINGUINE WITH ARUGULA PESTO

Time 30 min

ingredients

4 people

400 g of long pasta such as linguine

160 g of cleaned rocket

140 g of burrata stracciatella

40 g of pine nuts

60 g grated parmesan

56 dried tomatoes in oil

extra virgin olive oil

salt and pepper

Preparation

Collect the rocket, parmesan, pine nuts, salt, pepper and 23 tablespoons of oil in the blender glass for the recipe for linguine with rocket pesto. Combine the legumes until you obtain a smooth pesto. Chop the dried tomatoes. Boil the linguine in boiling salted water, drain when al dente and season with the pesto, adding, if necessary, a spoonful of cooking water until you obtain a creamy sauce. Arrange the linguine on plates, complete with the chopped dried tomatoes and serve immediately.

BEAN AND CHESTNUT SOUP

Time 40 minutes

ingredients

4 people

250 g of borlotti beans

250 g of boiled chestnuts

100 g 1 slice of bacon

Pepper powder

homemade bread

extra virgin olive oil

salt, garlic

Preparation

For the bean and chestnut soup recipe, boil the beans for about an hour and 20 minutes, turn off the heat and season with salt. Let them rest for 5 minutes. Brown 1 whole clove of peeled garlic in a pan with a drizzle of extra virgin olive oil. Add the diced bacon with a little pepper powder and fry for 3 minutes. Add the boiled chestnuts to the bean casserole, heat and cook together for 10 minutes, then add the browned bacon. Serve the soup accompanied with toasted croutons. You can garnish, if you like, with aromatic herbs such as sage or bay leaves.

HALF SLEEVES WITH WHITE SAUCE AND WALNUTS

Time 17 min

ingredients

4 people

320 g type of short pasta

short sleeves

80 g of milk

80 g of walnut kernels plus some

3 anchovy fillets in oil

1 pear, garlic

butter, salt, pepper

extra virgin olive oil

Preparation

For the recipe for mezze sleeves with bechamel and walnuts, boil the water for the pasta. In the meantime, prepare the sauce: blend 60 g of walnuts with the milk, anchovies, 30 g of oil and a clove of garlic with an immersion blender. Salt the water and throw in the pasta. While it is cooking, clean the pear without peeling it and cut it into chunks. Brown them in a pan with a knob of butter for 3 minutes. Dilute the sauce with a ladle of pasta cooking water. Drain the pasta, toss it in the pan with the pears, adding the sauce. Complete with pepper and the remaining kernels.

RED SPAGHETTI WITH GARLIC, OIL AND CHILI PEPPER

Time 50 min

ingredients

4 people

800 g of beets

350 grams of spaghetti

1 clove of garlic

1 fresh chili pepper

whole yogurt

chives, parsley

extra virgin olive oil

coarse and fine salt

pepper

Preparation

For the recipe for red spaghetti with garlic, oil and chilli pepper, peel the beets and extract the juice with the extractor (alternatively blend the beetroot pulp with 1.5 liters of water and then filter the juice). Dry the extraction waste in the microwave, spreading it well on a plate. It will take at least 8 minutes. Check every 12 minutes to prevent the powder from burning. Brown 1 sliced clove of garlic and 1 sliced fresh chili pepper in a pan in 34 tablespoons of oil for a couple of minutes.

Add the spaghetti, a pinch of coarse salt and toast the pasta briefly like a risotto. Start pouring hot water, then add a little beetroot juice and continue alternating the two liquids until the spaghetti is cooked. Season 4 tablespoons of yogurt with salt, oil and the chopped chives. Distribute the spaghetti on plates and complete with the yogurt sauce, garlic slices, parsley leaves and pepper.

SMOKED RISOTTO WITH CHESTNUTS

Time 50 minutes

ingredients

4 people

1 kg of fresh chestnuts

250 g of Carnaroli rice

250 g of butter

Grana Padano Dop

ground coffee

shells, sea urchins and leaves

of chestnuts

lemon, salt

Preparation

For the recipe for smoked risotto with chestnuts, remove the peel from the chestnuts and boil them for 10 minutes (still steam a little); finally peel them, saving the shells for smoking the butter. You will need to obtain 200 g of clean boiled chestnuts. Smoke the butter: Place a generous handful of shells and sea urchins in a large saucepan, turn the heat on high and then turn it off to create smoke. Overlay a sieve, lined with baking paper, and distribute 120 g of diced butter: the butter must be very cold or frozen so that it does not melt, and that the cubes are not too large;

close the lid and leave to smoke for about ten minutes; the butter fat will absorb the flavor molecules from the smoke. Dry toast the rice with 1 teaspoon of salt; after 1 minute start cooking it by wetting it with boiling water; when it is still al dente, add the chestnuts, 4 tablespoons of grated parmesan and 125 g of smoked butter, adding more boiling water little by little to adjust the consistency, which should be soft; finally add 23 tablespoons of lemon juice. Serve the risotto as soon as it is ready, completing with a light sprinkling of coffee and grated boiled chestnuts.

SPAGHETTONI WITH CASHEW AND PEPPER

Time 35 min

ingredients

4 people

380 grams of spaghetti

70 g of natural cashews

70 g nutritional yeast flakes

miso

black peppercorns

extra virgin olive oil

salt

Preparation

For the cashew and pepper spaghetti recipe, place the cashews in a high-powered blender with the yeast flakes, 2 tablespoons of miso and 2 tablespoons of water. Toast 1 tablespoon of peppercorns in a small pan, then crush them in the mortar or with a meat tenderizer, between two sheets of baking paper. Boil the spaghetti in boiling salted water; drain them 2 minutes before the end, directly in the pan with the cashew cream; finish cooking them with a little of their cooking water. Serve them with freshly ground pepper and a drizzle of oil.

RED CABBAGE RISOTTO AND PARMESAN FONDUE

Time 90 min

ingredients

4 people

800 g 1 red cabbage

320 grams of rice

90 g grated parmesan

50 g of shelled walnuts

30 g of butter, 30 g of milk

3 stalks of celery

3 onions, 2 carrots

1 shallot, salt

dry white wine

extra virgin olive oil

Preparation

For the red cabbage risotto and parmesan fondue recipe, prepare the vegetable broth: put the celery, carrots and 2 onions in a saucepan with 2 liters of water, lightly salt and cook for at least 1 hour. Finally filtered back into the saucepan. Quickly toast the shelled walnuts; as soon as they are slightly golden, remove them and set them aside. Peel the cabbage, cut the leaves into strips and simmer them in a saucepan with 1 small chopped onion, salt and broth, adding as it dries; when the cabbage is tender, blend and then filter it through a fine mesh strainer until you obtain a smooth cream. Chop the shallot and sauté it in a saucepan in a drizzle of oil, then add the rice and toast it until it is very hot; then blend with the white wine. Then proceed by wetting it little by little with a little boiling broth; halfway through cooking, mix with a few spoonfuls of cabbage cream and finish cooking. In the meantime, pour the milk into a saucepan, bring it almost to the boil, turn off the heat, add 60 g of grated parmesan, and mix carefully to mix the ingredients well; keep this sauce hot in a sweet bain-marie. Stir the risotto with the butter and the rest of the parmesan; cover it with the lid and let it rest for a few minutes. Finally, distribute on a serving platter or individual plates and complete with the parmesan fondue and crumbled toasted walnuts.

TURNIP TOPS AND LEMON RISOTTO

Time 50 minutes

ingredients

4 people servings

360 g of Carnaroli rice

250 g of turnip greens

80 g butter, garlic

80 g parmesan

20 g acacia honey, 1 chilli pepper

12 whole leaves of turnip greens

untreated lemon

vegetable broth,

extra virgin olive oil

salt and pepper

Preparation

For the risotto with turnip greens and lemon recipe, collect 200 g of lemon juice in a saucepan and reduce it by a third. Add the honey and let it melt. Leave to cool, then add 150 g of extra virgin olive oil and whip with an immersion blender, obtaining a sauce. Blanch the whole turnip top leaves, then drain them, dry them and arrange them on a plate covered with cling film and greased with oil. Cover with additional cling film, prick holes and place in the microwave until the leaves are crisp. Peel the turnip tops and blanch them in boiling salted water, cool them in water and ice, then drain them and squeeze them lightly. Brown them in a pan with a drizzle of oil, 1 clove of garlic and 1 chili pepper, for 12 minutes. Drain the excess oil, remove the garlic and chilli and blend them, adding some vegetable broth until you obtain a cream. Toast the rice in a saucepan with a pinch of salt, blend and bring to the boil, adding the vegetable broth little by little (about 1.5 litres). 1 minute before the end of cooking, add the turnip greens cream and mix. Stir the risotto with the butter, a drizzle of oil, the parmesan, salt and pepper. Serve it with the lemon sauce and garnished with the crispy leaves and grated lemon zest.

ORECCHIETTE, TURNIP TOPS AND GINGER

Time 25 min

ingredients

4 people

500 g of fresh orecchiette

320 g of cleaned turnip greens

garlic

fresh ginger

extra virgin olive oil

salt

pepper

Preparation

For the orecchiette, turnip tops and ginger recipe, blanch the turnip tops in boiling salted water for 30 seconds and drain them with a slotted spoon. Boil the orecchiette in the same water as the turnip tops. Chop the tops and brown them in a pan with 3 tablespoons of oil, 1 clove of garlic and 1 teaspoon of grated ginger. When they start to sizzle, wet them with 1 ladle of the pasta cooking water. Drain the orecchiette and season them directly in the pan with the tops, completing with freshly ground pepper.

SPAGHETTI WITH COD SAUCE

Time 60 min

ingredients

4 people servings

400 g of peeled tomatoes

350 grams of spaghetti

350 g of cod, soaked and desalted

4 bran peppers

3 shallots, 1 egg

small salted capers

re-milled durum wheat semolina

extra virgin olive oil

white wine, salt

Preparation

For the spaghetti with cod sauce recipe, finely slice the shallot and simmer it gently in a pan with a drizzle of oil; then blend with 1/2 glass of wine, then add the roughly chopped tomatoes and cook the sauce over low heat for 30 minutes. Cut the cabbage into 45cm slices. Dip in the beaten egg, then in the durum wheat semolina, and fry in plenty of oil. Add the cod and capers to the sauce and cook for another 30 minutes. Boil the spaghetti in plenty of salted water. Drain them al dente, using the appropriate ladle, directly into the saucepan and finish cooking, adding a drop of the cooking water if necessary. Fry the brain peppers for 30 seconds in plenty of boiling oil. Drain them, crumble them over the pasta and serve.

AUTUMN PORRIDGE

Time 80 min

ingredients

4 people

200 g of fresh porcini mushrooms

150 g of boiled lentils

100 g of wholemeal oat flakes

garlic, rosemary, sage

dry bay leaf

soy sauce

vegetables for the broth

fennel beards

extra virgin olive oil

White pepper

black peppercorns

Preparation

For the autumn porridge recipe, clean the porcini mushrooms and cut them into pieces. Save the discarded stem parts, clean the soil, and collect in a saucepan with 12 liters of water, vegetable broth, according to your onion remains, and 1 celery stalk. Scented with sage leaves, 1 sprig of rosemary, dried bay leaves and black peppercorns. Simmer for 1 hour, then strain. Brown the porcini mushrooms in a pan with a drizzle of oil, 1 clove of garlic with the peel and 1 sprig of rosemary, browning them for 3 minutes. Add a splash of soy sauce and a grind of white pepper. Toast the oat flakes in a saucepan, dry, until hot:

touching them will have to burn, and it will take 23 minutes. Pour the broth until it generously covers the oats and cook it for about 1015 minutes, like a risotto, i.e. add the broth little by little as it is absorbed. Also add the lentils and half the mushrooms, browned for 2 minutes before turning off, then stir in 23 tablespoons of oil and leave to rest. Serve the porridge complete with the remaining roasted mushrooms and sprigs of fennel beard.

SPAGHETTI WITH PORCINI AND PECORINO

Time 25 min

ingredients

4 servings

350 grams of spaghetti

100 g of pecorino

4 porcini mushroom caps

extra virgin olive oil

salt

peppercorns

Preparation

For the spaghetti with pecorino recipe, heat the water in a large pan and, when it boils, add salt and add the spaghetti. In the meantime, clean the porcini mushroom caps and cut them into slices. In a pan, dry toast some ground pepper, add a drizzle of oil, the porcini mushrooms and sauté for 2 minutes; then pour in 1 ladle of pasta cooking water and cook for another 1 minute. Collect the pecorino in a bowl and mix it with 1 ladle of pasta water to create a sauce. Drain the spaghetti al dente directly into the pan with the mushrooms and add a little more water to complete cooking. Remove from the heat, add the pecorino sauce, mix well and serve.

VALPELLINESE SOUP

Time 60 minutes

ingredients

4 people servings

600 grams of cabbage

400 g of meat broth

400 g of rye bread

300 g Fontina cheese

150 grams of butter

100 grams of bacon

1 egg, salt,

and pepper

Preparation

For the Zuppa alla Valpellinese recipe, blend the bread with the fontina cheese with the food processor. Also add the egg, salt and pepper and mix until you obtain a homogeneous mixture. Form these into balls, as big as olives. Clean the cabbage and cut it into strips, keeping 2 whole leaves aside for decoration. Melt 100 g of butter in a saucepan together with the lard. When they have melted, add the strips of cabbage and let them flavour, stirring; close with the lid and leave to cook for about 56 minutes. Then add the broth and cook for another 20 minutes.

In the meantime, brown the bread and cheese balls in a pan with 50 g of butter for about 56 minutes. Add them to the cabbage casserole and cook everything together for another 10/12 minutes. Toast the cabbage leaves kept aside in the microwave: spread them on the tray and cook in the microwave at maximum power for 7/8 minutes, for 30 seconds at a time, turning the leaves at each interval. Serve the soup with balls of bread and fontina and dried cabbage leaves.

PISAREI AND FAŚÖ DI PIACENZA

Time 1h

ingredients

68 people

300 g of boiled beans

50 g of bacon, 1 carrot

1 stalk of celery

half an onion, parsley

bay leaf, garlic

butter, salt

extra virgin olive oil

for Pisarei

200 g of breadcrumbs

200 g of flour

extra virgin olive oil

salt, bay leaf, black pepper

extra virgin olive oil

Preparation

Peel and chop the celery, carrot and onion. Sauté them in a non-stick saucepan with 3 tablespoons of oil and 1/2 tablespoon of butter, together with 1 crushed garlic clove with its peel and a sprig of parsley leaves. Add the boiled beans, the bacon cut into pieces and 1 bay leaf and brown them together with the sauté until they almost start to stick to the pan a little: you should smell a toasted, almost burnt aroma. Add salt and water until the beans are generously covered. Bring to the boil, cover with a lid and cook for about 1 hour. for the pisarei, bring about 300 g of water to the boil. Pour it several times onto the breadcrumbs, season with 1 tablespoon of oil and a pinch of salt. Knead (the amount of water can vary depending on the quality of the breadcrumbs, more or less dry), until you obtain a dough, then add the flour. Collect it in a loaf and let it rest covered for 30 minutes. Form many small loaves (about ø 5 mm) with the dough, then detach small portions and make the pisarei by digging out the pieces of dough with your thumb on the pastry board. Remove the garlic clove and bay leaf from the bean casserole, add the pisarei and cook for about 5 minutes. Turn off the heat and let it rest with the lid, like a risotto, to concentrate all the aromas. Serve them on a plate, completing them with fresh bay leaves, a drizzle of raw oil and ground black pepper.

LASAGNA WITH AUTUMN VEGETABLES

Time 1h 10 min

ingredients

4 people

1 liter bechamel

500 g of flour

200 g of cleaned pumpkin

200 g of cleaned celeriac

200 g of carrots, 5 eggs

Grated parmesan

extra virgin olive oil

salt and pepper

Preparation

For the lasagna recipe with autumn vegetables, mix the flour and eggs in the planetary mixer. Let the dough rest covered for 30 minutes. Using the vegetable chopper, slice the pumpkin and celeriac and grate the carrots. Fry the vegetables with oil, salt and pepper. Roll out the dough with the sheeter to 1 mm. Make the lasagna by alternating the pasta with the béchamel sauce, the vegetables and the parmesan. Bake at 180°C for about 20 minutes.

SPINACH SOUP

Time 30 min

ingredients

4 servings

650 g of potatoes

300 g of almond milk

unsweetened

250 g of new spinach

200 g of spicy sausage

with pepper and fennel

80 g of spring onions

40 g of almonds in their skin

extra virgin olive oil, salt

Preparation

For the spinach soup recipe, chop the spring onions and fry them in a saucepan with 1 tablespoon of oil; add the peeled potatoes cut into thin slices, 300 g of water and the almond milk; cook for 15 minutes. Add the spinach, salt, cook for another 5 minutes, then blend everything until you obtain a cream. Shell the sausage and toast. Cut the almonds into slices and toast them. Serve the cream with the sausage and almonds. Garnish to taste with baby spinach leaves, a drizzle of oil and freshly ground black pepper.

RECIPES
SECOND DISHES

STEAMED FISH FILLET WITH HERBS

Preparation time: 10 minutes

Cooking time: 15 minutes

Servings: 4

Ingredients:

4 white fish fillets

(for example, cod or cod)

Juice of half a lemon

2 cloves of garlic

Chopped fresh parsley

Extra virgin olive oil

Salt and pepper to taste

Preparation

Marinate the fish: In a bowl, marinate the fish fillets with lemon juice, chopped garlic, parsley, oil, salt and pepper. Leave to marinate for at least 15 minutes. Steam: Place the marinated fillets in a steamer basket. Cook for about 15 minutes, or until the fish is cooked through and flakes with a fork. Tips: Fish: You can replace white fish with other types of fish, such as salmon or trout.

TURKEY AND COURGETTE MEATBALLS

Preparation time: 20 minutes

Cooking time: 20 minutes

Servings: 4

Ingredients:

500g of ground turkey

1 courgette

1 egg

50g of breadcrumbs

Grated parmesan

Chopped fresh parsley

Garlic powder

Salt and pepper to taste

Extra virgin olive oil

Preparation

Prepare the vegetables: Grate the courgette. Mix the ingredients: In a bowl, combine the ground turkey, grated courgette, egg, breadcrumbs, parmesan, parsley, garlic powder, salt and pepper. Mix well until you obtain a homogeneous mixture. Shape the meatballs: With slightly damp hands, shape the meatballs. Cook the meatballs: In a pan, heat a drizzle of oil and cook the meatballs over medium heat until they are golden on all sides.

VALDOSTANE CUTLETS

Time 40 min

ingredients

6 people

600 g of veal slices

200 g Fontina cheese

150 g of sliced cooked ham

140 grams of butter

2 eggs

bread crumbs

salt

Preparation

For the Valle d'Aosta cutlets recipe, beat the veal slices and cut them into a rectangular shape. Divide the fontina into six slices. Place a slice of fontina cheese and a slice of ham on each slice of meat, then close it. Dip the stuffed meat first in the lightly beaten eggs and then in the breadcrumbs, repeating the operation a second time to seal the cutlets well. Heat half the butter in a pan until foamy, and cook the first 3 cutlets over medium heat for a couple of minutes on each side. Throw away the used butter and repeat the operation with the other half of the butter to cook the three remaining cutlets. Dry the cutlets on kitchen paper, salt them and serve hot.

RABBIT ROASTS WITH SAEURIER AND SPECK AND APPLE CREAM WITH MUSTARD

Time 1h 30 min

ingredients

4 people

Mustard apple cream pearl

230 g of apple juice

20 g of mustard syrup

2.5 g of agaragar

For roasts

385 g 1 box of sauerkraut

180 g Speck Alto Adige

50 g parmesan, 4 rabbit legs

thyme, garlic, rosemary

extra virgin olive oil

salt and pepper

Preparation

For the apple mustard cream, heat the apple juice and mustard syrup with the agar agar and cook for 6 minutes after boiling. Turn it off, let it cool, cover it with cling film and put it in the fridge for 1 hour, until you get a jelly. For roasts, debone the rabbit legs. Rinse the sauerkraut and season it with a drizzle of oil, salt and pepper. Stuff the rabbit legs with sauerkraut and close, trying to recompose the shape of the leg. Then wrap them in slices of speck, so as to cover them entirely and seal any openings. Place the roasts obtained in a baking dish, and season them with oil, salt and pepper;

add a few sprigs of thyme and rosemary and 1 clove of garlic to the pan. Bake at 160°C for about 45 minutes. Create a disk with 2 tablespoons of grated parmesan on a sheet of baking paper and cook it in the microwave at maximum power for 2 minutes. Place the waffle on a curved surface and let it cool. Prepare another one in the same way. Serve the roasts with the apple cream, softened with a whisk, and the chopped parmesan wafers.

BAKED CHICKEN WITH LEMON, ORANGES AND LAURLES DRESS

Time 1h 20min

ingredients

4 people

2 chickens (600 g each)

1 lemon

1 orange

Bay leaves

fresh cream

extra virgin olive oil

salt

Preparation

Pass the chickens over the flame to remove any remaining feathers. Massage the skin with 2 tablespoons of cream (alternatively, with a knob of butter). Insert 2 bay leaves and half the orange and lemon peels into each chicken. Sprinkle with a little salt, place them on an oiled baking tray and bake at 200°C for 10 minutes. Remove the chickens from the oven, let them cool for 5 minutes, then cover them with thinly cut citrus fruit slices (3 mm) alternating with bay leaves, with the bottom part facing up, until the entire top part is covered. Tie them with string or use the most convenient roasting net on the market. Return the chicken to the pan, season each with a pinch of salt and a few tablespoons of oil, and bake again at 200°C for 4050 minutes, until the skin is golden.

AROMATIC FISH WITH PAPRIKA, TURMERIC AND CITRUS

Time 30 min

ingredients

6 people

250 g 4 sea bream fillets

260 g 2 sea bass fillets

250 g 2 sea bream fillets

1 lime

1 bergamot

1 grapefruit, salt

turmeric, sweet paprika

extra virgin olive oil

Preparation

For the recipe of aromatic fish with paprika, turmeric and citrus fruits, clean the fish fillets by removing the bones with tweezers. Heat a non-stick pan very vigorously, then place the fish fillets in it, two at a time, skin side down, keeping it adherent to the bottom for 1 minute, until it starts to release its juices; remove the fillets from the heat and remove the skin. Finally, season them with a drizzle of oil, then with a pinch of salt, on both sides. Sprinkle the sea bream fillets on the meat side (the one opposite to the one where the skin was) with 1 teaspoon of turmeric; Use a fine mesh strainer to better distribute the powder. Proceed in the same way, sprinkling the sea bass with 1 teaspoon of paprika. Mix the grated zest of 1 lime, ½ bergamot and 1/3 grapefruit in a bowl. Avoid grating the white part (albedo) which would give a bitter taste.

Sprinkle the sea bream fillets, always on the meat side, with this peel mixture. Cook the fish fillets, two at a time, in a very hot pan, first on the side with the aromas for a few seconds and then for 12 minutes on the other side, the one where the skin was. Alternatively you can cook the fish in a pan in the oven at 200°C for about ten minutes. It is important to cook the fish in the following order: first the sea bream fillets with turmeric, then the sea bass with citrus fruits and finally the sea bass with paprika, so as not to alter the colours. Always use a spatula to move the fillets so as not to break them.

MAMMOLESE STOCK

Time 45 min

ingredients

4 people servings

1 kg of soaked stockfish

1 kg of potatoes

600 g of peeled tomatoes or sauce

3 chillies

2 red onions

pitted olives in brine

salted capers

extra virgin olive oil

salt

Preparation

For the mammolese stockfish recipe, peel the potatoes and divide each one into 4 wedges. In a saucepan (preferably earthenware) fry the sliced onions with 5 tablespoons of oil for 23 minutes; add the tomato and cook for 5 minutes, season with salt. Add the potatoes and continue cooking for 78 minutes, adding a ladle of water if the sauce dries out. Add the stockfish cut into pieces, 3 tablespoons of olives, 1 tablespoon of desalted capers, the chillies and continue cooking for 20 minutes, stirring occasionally, until the potatoes are cooked. Serve the stockfish flavored to taste with fresh thyme leaves.

POACHED EGG ON SWEET AND SOUR ESCAROLE

Time 40 min

ingredients

4 people servings

100 g of pine nuts

100 g of red wine

80 g of raisins

20 grams of butter

4 eggs

2 heads of escarole

1 onion

extra virgin olive oil

vinegar, salt, pepper

Preparation

For the poached egg on sweet and sour
escarole recipe, sauté the escarole with a
little oil and salt, with the lid on over low
heat, for 78 minutes. Cut the onion into slices
and brown it in another saucepan with a
drizzle of oil and salt. Add the red wine and
cook uncovered until all the liquid has
evaporated. Mix the onion with the escarole,
raisins and pine nuts and toast them quickly
in a pan (let them brown without chopping
them). Prepare the poached eggs: bring
unsalted water to the boil, acidulated with a
splash of vinegar; shell one egg at a time into
a saucer and slide it into the center of a
vortex created in the water with a spoon.
Cook it for 45 minutes, then drain it;
proceed like this with the remaining eggs.
Serve them on the escarole and season with
salt and pepper.

ORANGE SALMON MEATBALLS

Time 1h

ingredients

4 people

500 g salmon steak

500 g of broccoli

300 g of breadcrumbs

30 g grated parmesan

3 eggs

2 untreated oranges

1 untreated lemon

chopped parsley

fresh ginger

fresh rosemary

dry white wine

extra virgin olive oil

salt, garlic

Preparation

For the orange salmon meatballs recipe, cook the salmon in the oven at 170°C for 1520 minutes. Remove the skin and any bones and crumble into a bowl. Mix with the eggs, then add some parsley, 1 teaspoon grated ginger, 150g breadcrumbs, parmesan and salt. Let the mixture rest in the fridge for 20 minutes. Meanwhile, blanch the broccoli in boiling salted water for 30 seconds. Drain them with a slotted spoon into a large bowl with water and ice and let them cool. Place the broccoli in boiling water and continue cooking for 1015 minutes. Drain them and keep them aside. Grate the zest of 1 orange. Squeeze the juice and mix it with 1/2 glass of white wine.

Peel the other orange, i.e. also removing the white part of the zest and the peel; divide it into pieces. Shape the salmon mixture with slightly damp hands into meatballs; pass them in the remaining breadcrumbs. Brown 23 cloves of garlic in a pan, remove them and arrange the meatballs (a few at a time) and 1 sprig of rosemary. Brown them over high heat for 23 minutes per side or until they are golden. Add the white wine and orange juice, lower the heat and finish cooking for another 34 minutes. Finally add the pieces of orange. Fry the broccoli in a pan with hot oil and 2 cloves of garlic. Season with salt, turn off the heat and add the grated orange zest. Serve the meatballs with the broccoli.

TURBOT OF FILLET WITH CALVADOS AND LEEK CREAM WITH PAPRIKA

Time 45 min

ingredients

4 people

1.5 kg turbot fillets

500 g of vegetable broth

3 apples, 2 leeks

1 small potato

sweet paprika

Calvados apple distillate

Marjoram

extra virgin olive oil

salt and pepper

Preparation

For the recipe for turbot fillet with calvados and leek cream with paprika, peel the potato and 1 apple and cut them into small pieces; cut the leeks into slices, eliminating the green part. Heat 4 tablespoons of oil in a pan and brown the potato, apple and leek for 12 minutes; add the vegetable broth and cook for 25 minutes, season with salt. Add 1 tablespoon of sweet paprika and blend everything with an immersion blender, obtaining a cream. Heat a drizzle of oil in a pan and cook the turbot fillets on the meat side for 2 minutes; turn them, season with salt, sprinkle with a splash of Calvados and continue cooking for another 45 minutes. Cut the other 2 apples into thin slices, removing the central part with the core. Remove the skin from the turbot fillets and serve them with leek cream and sliced apples,

SMOKED MEAT

Time 25 min

ingredients

4 people servings

480 g 4 slices of roast beef

4 mandarins

1 head of late radicchio

1 bunch of rocket

1 head of Belgian endive

extra virgin olive oil

Rosemary

juniper berries

salt and pepper

Preparation

For the smoked meat recipe, season the slices
of roast beef with a drizzle of oil, a pinch of
salt, a grind of pepper, a sprig of rosemary
and a few juniper berries. Arrange them on
a plate and place a saucepan filled with
boiling water on top. Cook them, without the
lid, for 68 minutes. Turn them over and cook
for another 46 minutes (extend or reduce the
cooking time according to your taste).
Prepare a mixed salad with radicchio,
Belgian endive, rocket and a few slices of
peeled raw mandarin. Season with oil, salt
and mandarin juice.

PAN-FISHED SEABASS IN WINE

Time 25 min

ingredients

Portions for 2 people

600 g 1 sea bass

downsized and gutted

1 clove of garlic

lemon

parsley

Rosemary

wise

dry white wine

extra virgin olive oil

salt and pepper

Preparation

For the pan-fried sea bass in wine recipe, wash the sea bass inside and out, then dry it with kitchen paper. Salt and pepper the belly and insert the garlic clove cut in two, 1 sprig of rosemary, 2 pieces of lemon, 2 sage leaves and a drizzle of oil. Place the fish in a nonstick pan that fits snugly. Season it with a drizzle of oil and cook it over medium-low heat with a lid for 3 minutes. Wet with a touch of white wine, let it evaporate, then collect the sauce with a spoon and pour it over the fish. Cover again and cook for another 4 minutes. Gently turn the sea bass, using a spatula and a fork, cover and cook for another 67 minutes, adding another touch of wine halfway through cooking and basting with the sauce. Turn off the heat and serve the sea bass with raw oil and chopped parsley,

PORK ROUND WITH MILK AND ONIONS

Time 1h

ingredients

4 people servings

1 kg of pork loin

1 liter of milk

350 g of white onions

2 juniper berries

1 aromatic bunch

(sage, rosemary, bay leaf)

pepper, salt

extra virgin olive oil

Preparation

For the pork loin recipe with milk and onions, brown the loin for 1015 minutes in a saucepan covered in oil so that it browns on all sides. Transfer to a plate and brown the sliced onions in the same saucepan for 45 minutes. Add the meat, the bouquet garni, the juniper, the milk again and bring to the boil. Reduce the heat, add salt and pepper, cover and cook for at least 1 hour. Blend the onions and broth, slice the pork loin and serve with the creamy sauce, accompanied, if desired, by mashed potatoes.

CHICKEN NUGGETS WITH OATS

Time 35 min + 20 min rest

ingredients

2 people

300 g of chicken breast

80 g of breadsticks

3 slices of bread

2 eggs

1 orange

half a red onion

flour, salt

oat flakes

extra virgin olive oil

Preparation

For the recipe for chicken nuggets with oats, blend the breadsticks in a cutter with the grated zest of 1/2 orange, without reducing it to flour, but leaving the consistency a little coarse. Then add 2 tablespoons of oat flakes and give it another shot of the cutter. Pour this mixture into a baking dish and mix it with another 2 tablespoons of oat flour. Cut the chicken into small pieces, removing any impurities. Blend it too in the cutter with the onion peeled and cut into small pieces, the slices of bread without the crust, 2 tablespoons of oil and a pinch of salt. Leave the mixture to rest for 1520 minutes, then form 6 round croquettes, slightly flattened.

Dip in the flour, then in the well beaten eggs, and finally in the mixture of breadsticks and oat flakes. Cook the chicken nuggets in a pan with a drizzle of not too hot extra virgin olive oil, leaving them to brown for at least 3 minutes on each side, so that they are golden on the outside and cooked on the inside too. Alternatively, season them with a drizzle of oil, place them on a baking tray and bake at 180°C for about 20 minutes. Serve with salad and ketchup-like sauce, if desired.

CACCIATORE-STYLE TUNA

Time 30 min

ingredients

24 people

500 g fresh tuna steak

100 g of mixed salad

30 g of pitted green olives

corn starch

Rosemary

fennel

untreated lemon

balsamic vinegar

Red wine

extra virgin olive oil

salt, pepper, garlic

Preparation

For the tuna hunter recipe, finely chop 1/2 clove of garlic. Brown the tuna over high heat in a hot pan for 3 minutes on one side, with salt and pepper. Turn and brown the other side too, with salt and pepper. Also burn it a little on the sides, just to color it. To obtain a regular tile you need to trim: in this case the doses will only be enough for two or three people. Add the chopped garlic and immediately blend with 1 glass of red wine and 3 tablespoons of balsamic vinegar. Add the olives, always over high heat.

Continue cooking for another 6/7 minutes, turning the steak from time to time so that it browns well on both sides. Remove tuna from pan; add 1 scant teaspoon of corn starch to the sauce in the pan and dissolve immediately and quickly so as not to form lumps. Allow the cooking juices to thicken for 23 minutes over medium heat: it must not be too small. Season the mixed salad with salt, a drizzle of oil, a few drops of lemon and the grated zest. Serve the tuna piping hot, sprinkled with its sauce and accompanied by the salad.

SEAFOOD SOUP
WITH CELERIAC

Time 60 min

ingredients

4 people

1 monkfish fillet

100 g clams

8 scampi

2 medium-sized cuttlefish

1 large celeriac

1 onion, 1 carrot

extra virgin olive oil

dry white wine

cumin, salt

black pepper, marjoram

Preparation

Clean the celeriac, cut it into slices about 1 cm thick and cut out 12 discs (ø 5 cm). Collect all the scraps in a pan, cover them with water and cook them for 30 minutes. Finally, blend by adding ½ teaspoon of cumin seeds and the cooking water until you obtain a soft cream. Place the celeriac discs in a pan with a drizzle of oil, salt and pepper. Bake in the oven at 180°C for 57 minutes. Cut the monkfish meat into large pieces (3 cm). Clean the scampi and cuttlefish. To tenderize the cuttlefish, make diagonal incisions on the bags. Prepare a fish broth (cardboard): in a pan, heat the onion and carrot pieces with a drizzle of oil,

brown the fish scraps, add 1 glass of wine
and add 1 liter of water. Cook over high heat
to reduce the liquid by half. Brown the
monkfish and clams in a large saucepan,
deglaze with ½ glass of wine, add the fish
broth and cover to open the shells. Drain the
freshly opened clams and keep them aside.
Cook over high heat to reduce the cooking
liquid by half. Finally, add the cuttlefish,
scampi and clams to the monkfish, sauté
everything for a few moments and turn off
the heat. Arrange the celeriac cream, the fish
and the celeriac slices on the plates and
complete with a drizzle of oil and marjoram
leaves.

FILLETS OF SOLE WITH POTATOES AND LEEK CREAM

Time 1h

ingredients

4 people servings

600 g of cleaned sole fillets

400 g 4 potatoes

200 g of cleaned leeks

150 g of breadcrumbs

40 g of dry white wine

garlic, parsley

extra virgin olive oil

salt and pepper

Preparation

For the sole fillets with potatoes and leek soup recipe, cut the leek into slices and place them in a saucepan with a drizzle of oil. Drain them and let them dry gently for 10 minutes. Peel a potato and cut it into chunks. Deglaze the leeks with the white wine, then add the diced potatoes, slowly add the water and cook over medium heat for 2025 minutes. In the meantime, peel the other potatoes and cut them into strips. Place them on a baking tray covered with baking paper. Season them with a drizzle of oil, salt and pepper and bake at 220°C for 30 minutes.

Blend the breadcrumbs with a sprig of parsley leaves, a clove of garlic and a pinch of salt until it becomes light green. Pass the sole fillets to cover them, then thread them onto 4 skewers, place them on a baking tray, on baking paper, and sprinkle them with more breadcrumbs. Blend the leeks with 2 tablespoons of oil, salt and pepper, obtaining a creamy soup. Remove the potato slices from the oven. Grease the sole fillets with a drizzle of oil and place them in the oven for 67 minutes. Serve them with potato strips and leek cream.

**BAKED TURBOT,
SOUR TURNIPES
ROASTED MANGO**

Time 50 min

ingredients

4 people

1 filleted turbot

2 yellow turnips, 2 red turnips

2 mangoes

1 carrot, 1 onion

cane sugar

dry white wine

rice vinegar

fresh mustard leaves

salt, sparkling water

extra virgin olive oil

Preparation

Heat a pan covered in oil, brown the diced onion and carrot, add the dry white wine. Allow to evaporate, continue to brown over high heat for 5 minutes, then add 1 liter of water. Season with salt and leave on the heat until the comic has reduced by half. Place the turbot fillets in a high-sided baking dish with a ladle of broth and bake at 180°C for 10 minutes. Clean the turnips, cut them into 45 mm cubes and soak them in cold water for a few minutes. Mix 10 g of brown sugar with 100 g of wine, 70 g of rice vinegar, a pinch of salt and 23 tablespoons of sparkling water in a bowl. Use part of the sauce to sauté first the yellow and striped turnips, then the red ones, in a hot pan for 5 minutes. Cut the central part of the mango pulp into cubes. Toast the garnishes over high heat in a very hot pan with a thin layer of oil and blend until you obtain a sauce. Arrange the cubes and mango sauce on plates, arrange the turbot fillets, turnips and a few leaves of fresh mustard.

SQUID STUFFED WITH CITRUS FRUIT

Time 1h

ingredients

4 people

50 g of breadcrumbs

50 g of shelled almonds

4 medium calamari

4 medium oranges

2 slices of bread

1 lemon, garlic

salted capers

parsley

Marjoram

extra virgin olive oil

salt and pepper

Preparation

For the citrus stuffed squid recipe, clean the squid and cut the tentacles into small pieces. Chop the almonds with a mixer or by placing them in a bag and crushing them with a meat mallet. Chop 2 small cloves of garlic and a sprig of parsley, place them in a pan with the chopped tentacles, 25 g of oil, a pinch of salt and freshly ground pepper and cook for 5 minutes. Chop the bread slices and mix them in a bowl with the chopped almonds, the breadcrumbs, the cooked tentacles, 2 tablespoons of unsalted capers, the juice of 1 and a half oranges, the grated lemon zest, a pinch of salt and a minced of pepper.

Stuff the squid with this filling, carefully distributing it into the bags; close them with a toothpick and place them on a baking tray lined with baking paper. Season them with oil, salt and pepper and bake at 180°C, in ventilated mode, for about 10 minutes; remove from the oven and moisten them with their cooking liquid and cook in the oven for another 510 minutes. Peel the remaining oranges, cut them into slices and season them with a drizzle of oil, a pinch of salt and a few leaves of marjoram. Serve the calamari with the orange salad.

SEABASS, MUSHROOMS, AND CERFOGLIO

Time 1h

ingredients

4 people

800 g of sea bass fillet

600 g chicken broth

200 g of porcini mushrooms

100 g of chervil

100 g of aubergines

5 g of brown sugar

2 red potatoes

2 spring onions, salt

thyme, garlic, shallot

extra virgin olive oil

Preparation

Blanch the chervil in boiling water and cool it in water and ice (reserve a few leaves for decoration). Chop 1 shallot and simmer it in a saucepan for 1 minute. Peel the potatoes and cut them into thin slices, add them to the shallots, add 200 g of chicken broth and cook for about 15 minutes. Let them cool, then blend them with the chervil until you obtain a smooth sauce. Pass it through a sieve for a more velvety consistency. Wash the aubergines and 200 g of porcini mushrooms. Cut them into cubes and sauté them separately in the pan until they are both golden: 45 minutes for the mushrooms, 67 minutes for the aubergines. In an oven-safe saucepan, brown the cleaned and chopped spring onions, add the mushrooms, aubergines and sugar.

Stir, add 400g chicken broth and bring to the boil. Cover the contents of the casserole with a sheet of wet and squeezed baking paper, in contact, and put the casserole in the oven for about 30 minutes at 140°C. Finally, blend without making the mixture too liquid, then pass through a sieve. Remove the caps from the black head porcini mushrooms and cut the stems into chunks. Brown everything in a pan with oil, thyme and 1 clove of garlic for 34 minutes. Scale and bone the fillet, then cut it into four portions, without peeling it. Season it with a drizzle of oil and drain it in a hot pan with a little salt on the bottom, placing it on the skin side. When the latter is crispy, transfer the slices to a baking tray lined with baking paper and finish cooking in the oven at 185°C for 5 minutes.

FISH STEW AND ZUCCHINI CREAM WITH SCAPECE

Time 1h 30min

ingredients

4 people

the courgette cream

250g chicken stock

5 courgettes, 1/2 shallot

potatoes, mint

white wine vinegar

extra virgin olive oil

salt and pepper

the stew

100 g of red mullet fillets

100 g of tuna fillet

100 g of sea bass fillets

4 scallops, 4 prawns

4 scampi, 4 clams

4 mussels, 1 clove of garlic

parsley, salt

extra virgin olive oil

Preparation

For the courgette cream, peel the courgettes, remove the part with the seeds and cut them into chunks. In a saucepan, fry the chopped shallot and a piece of finely chopped potato, add the courgettes and let them flavour. Douse them with a splash of vinegar, then add the hot chicken broth. Season with a few mint leaves and cook for 20 minutes. Blend everything, adding salt and pepper and adding 23 tablespoons of oil (for a greener sauce, peel the courgettes and blanch them the peels in boiling salted water; proceed with the recipe, cutting the peeled courgettes into cubes. When it's time to blend to obtain the sauce, add the blanched peels (if you want it very velvety, pass it through a sieve). For the stew, place the peeled garlic in a saucepan with a drizzle of oil and a little parsley. When the oil is hot, add the mussels and cover. Wet with a drop of water and cover again. Remove the mussels from the pan as soon as they open. Repeat the operation with the clams. Clean all the fish and cut them into small pieces. Shelled prawns, scampi and scallops. Drizzle them with a drizzle of oil and drain them for 34 minutes in a hot pan, sprinkled with a pinch of salt. Serve fish, molluscs and crustaceans in the courgette sauce, finished with fresh sprouts and raw oil if desired.

FISH WITH BREAD CRUMPS

Time 45 min

ingredients

4 people

500 g 4 fillets of

hake with skin

250 g of milk

60 g of breadcrumbs

20 g of flour

extra virgin olive oil

Marjoram

nutmeg

lemon, butter

salt and pepper

Preparation

For the breaded fish recipe, place the hake fillets on a large sheet of baking paper, and season them with 2 tablespoons of oil, salt, pepper and marjoram; close the bag and bake at 180°C for 2025 minutes. Once ready, remove from the oven and let it cool and finally remove the pulp in large pieces. In the meantime, prepare the béchamel: cook 20 g of butter with the flour, obtain a blonde mixture, add the cold milk, all at once, season with salt, pepper and nutmeg, and cook the béchamel for 34 minutes after having Remove from the boil, stirring continuously. Grease and cover a small baking tray with breadcrumbs; spread half the béchamel sauce on the bottom, add the fish, the grated lemon zest, the chopped marjoram, the breadcrumbs and the knobs of butter. Bake at 180°C for about 15 minutes. Serve with marjoram leaves.

FISH MEATLOAF WITH BROCCOLI, HERBS AROMATIC AND CREAM

Time 1h

ingredients

68 people

580 g of cleaned cod fillet

300 g of fresh cream

120 g of broccoli tufts

4 egg whites

coriander berries

chives, salt, dill

Preparation

For the fish meatloaf recipe with broccoli, aromatic herbs and cream, blanch the tufts

of broccoli in boiling salted water for 1 minute and drain. Clean the cod from any remaining bones, cut it into small pieces and add the cream, egg whites and a pinch of salt. Blend everything until you obtain a slightly sticky mass. Flavored with ground coriander and green pepper. Add the broccoli tufts to the mixture, after having dabbed them with kitchen paper, to dry them a little. Also, add a sprig of chopped dill along with some chives. Spread the mixture on a layer of overlapping sheets of foil suitable for cooking. Roll it up with the help of the film until you obtain a sausage. Tie it at the ends with kitchen string and steam the meatloaf for 45 minutes. serve it cut into slices. Accompany him as you like.

VEAL FILLET, APPLES AND CHICORY WITH PORT SAUCE

Time 1h 15min

ingredients

6 people servings

1.2kg clean veal fillet

and tied to the roast

250 g of red radicchio

30 g of butter, 4 g of corn starch

2 apples, 1 shallot

thyme, port wine

extra virgin olive oil

salt and pepper

Preparation

For the recipe for veal fillet, apples and radicchio with port, wash the apples and cut them into 8 segments. Heat a drizzle of oil in a pan, also suitable for the oven, brown the shallot cut in half, and toast the fillet on all sides for 5 minutes, adding salt and pepper, and flavoring with a sprig of thyme; add 1/2 glass of Port (about 80 g), let it evaporate for 1 minute, then transfer it to the oven and cook at 120°C for 15 minutes. Add the apples and continue cooking for another 40 minutes.

Transfer the fillet and apples to the serving tray and deglaze the pan with a glass of Port (about 150 g); let it evaporate, add 30 g of butter mixed with 4 g of corn starch, and cook for 3 minutes, then add 50 g of water, mix and cook for another 2 minutes, obtaining the sauce. Clean the radicchio and break it into pieces. Remove the string from the fillet, cut into medallions and serve with apples, radicchio and Porto sauce.

BORLOTTI MEATLOAF, GREEN BEANS AND CHEESE, WRAPPED IN HAM

Time 1h 30 min

ingredients

68 people

350 g of boiled borlotti beans

300 grams of potatoes

120 g of robiola type cheese

100 g of green beans

100 g of sliced raw ham

30 g parmesan

1 egg, marjoram

extra virgin olive oil

salt and pepper

Preparation

For the meatloaf recipe with borlotti beans, green beans and cheese wrapped in ham, boil the potatoes in boiling water for about 40 minutes. Clean the green beans and boil them in boiling salted water for 5 minutes, then drain them. Blend the beans with 3 tablespoons of oil using an immersion blender. Mash the potatoes and add them to the bean cream, together with the egg, grated parmesan, salt, pepper, a sprig of chopped marjoram and the chopped green beans. Mix everything until the ingredients are combined. Lay the ham slices next to each other on a sheet of baking paper, slightly overlapping each other.

You will obtain a rectangle: turn it so that the ham slices are vertical in front of you; arrange the meatloaf mixture on the base. Create a groove in the center and fill it with the cheese, then close the mixture giving it a cylindrical shape. Finally, roll it in the slices of ham, using the baking paper. Wrap the meatloaf in paper, as if it were a candy. Grease the outside with a drizzle of oil, place it in a baking dish and bake at 180°C for 35 minutes; then open the paper and cook for another 78 minutes.

GRATINATED COD

Time 50 min

ingredients

4 servings

800 g of desalted cod fillet

200 g of stale breadcrumbs

40 g of walnut kernels

40 g of raisins

8 dried figs

parsley, garlic

Red wine

extra virgin olive oil

Preparation

For the gratin cod recipe, clean the cod, remove all the bones and place it in a baking dish suitable for going from the oven to the table. Coarsely blend the breadcrumbs. Chop the figs, nuts and raisins. Finely chop a sprig of parsley with 1 clove of garlic and distribute part of it over the cod. Mix the remaining mixture with the breadcrumbs and the chopped dried fruit. Season the fish with a drizzle of red wine, then cover it with a mixture of bread and dried fruit. Season with a drizzle of oil and bake at 180°C for about 20 minutes.

CHICKEN AND PORCINI ROLLERS WITH GINGER IN KATAIFI PASTA

Time 40 min

ingredients

8 people

400 g 8 slices of chicken breast

180 g of porcini mushrooms

150 g of mayonnaise

125 g of Greek yogurt

90 g of bread for sandwiches

fresh ginger, salt

kataifi pasta

chives, basil

Peanut oil

extra virgin olive oil

Preparation

For the recipe for chicken, porcini and porcini mushroom rolls with ginger, in kataifi paste, remove the crust from the bread and blend it. Clean the mushrooms and cut them into small pieces. Brown in a pan with a drizzle of extra virgin olive oil, 34 slices of ginger and a pinch of salt for 23 minutes. Turn it off and let it cool. Finely chop the mushrooms, finely chop the browned ginger and add everything to the bread. Season with salt and add 1 tablespoon of sliced chives to this filling.

Lightly beat the chicken breast slices to thin them, fill them in the center with a knob of stuffing and close into a roll. Wrap each chicken roll in kataifi dough; fry them for 3 minutes in peanut oil at 170°C, with 23 slices of ginger. Drain them on kitchen paper. Mix the mayonnaise with the Greek yogurt, a small piece of grated ginger and a few chopped basil leaves. Serve the rolls with the ginger mayonnaise.

LUCIANA-STYLE FISHERMAN AND CRISPY ARTICHOKES

Time 1h 10min

ingredients

4 people servings

1kg monkfish slice

150 g of tomato puree

80 g of pitted green olives

30 g of desalted capers

3 artichokes

1 lemon

1 clove of garlic

Marjoram

thyme, bay leaf

celery salt

extra virgin olive oil

Peanut oil

Preparation

For the Luciana monkfish recipe, clean the monkfish slice and remove the cuticles; turn it over, make two incisions along the central bone, remove it and keep it aside. Tie the monkfish steak like a roast: in this way it will maintain greater succulence during cooking. Prepare an aromatic bouquet with a sprig of marjoram, a sprig of thyme, a couple of bay leaves and a stalk of celery. Heat a pan, preferably cast iron or steel, with 2 tablespoons of oil; brown the roasted monkfish for 1 minute, add salt, add the peeled and crushed garlic and the aromatic bunch, the olives and the desalted capers,

then cover everything with the tomato puree;
add 50 g of water, and the monkfish bone,
cover and cook for 50 minutes over low heat.
Clean the artichokes, eliminating the thorns
and the internal beard; cut them into wedges
and gradually immerse them in water
acidulated with lemon juice. Fry the
artichokes in plenty of peanut oil for 56
minutes, then drain them on kitchen paper
and sabatelli. Slice the roasted monkfish and
serve it with its sauce and crunchy
artichokes.

SCALLOPS WITH GRAPES AND MUSHROOMS

Time 20 min

ingredients

4 people

300 g of fresh porcini mushrooms

120 g of seedless white grapes

120 g of seedless red grapes

12 scallop nuts

butter, garlic

parsley

salt and pepper

Preparation

For the scallops with grapes and mushrooms recipe, roast the scallops in a pan, in a knob of foaming butter, over high heat, turning them on both sides, for 23 minutes. Salt them lightly. Transfer the shellfish to a plate and keep the cooking juices. Clean the baking tray with kitchen paper. Clean the mushrooms and cut them into small pieces. Cut the larger grapes in half. Add a new knob of butter to the pan and sauté the porcini mushrooms and grapes with 1 crushed garlic clove and a pinch of salt for 3 minutes. Put the scallops and their cooking juices back in the pan, mix, remove the garlic and pepper and serve with chopped parsley.

FANS WITH PORCINI AND POTATOES

Time 1h

ingredients

6 servings

6 small yellow potatoes

150 g of porcini mushrooms

30 g parmesan

2 pieces of shallots

laurel, wise

marten, salty

Rosemary

red wine, butter

tomato paste

extra virgin olive oil

salt and pepper

Preparation

For the potato flan recipe, peel the potatoes and wash them in a bowl until the water runs clear, to remove some of the starch. Cut the potatoes into regular slices 34 mm thick. Massage them with a drizzle of oil, spread on a baking tray lined with baking paper and salt them lightly. Clean the porcini mushrooms, cut them into regular slices, distribute them in the pan with the potatoes, and season them with a drizzle of oil. Bake at 220°C for 15 minutes. Butter 6 muffin molds (ø 7 cm) and line the bottom with 6 discs of baking paper, which should also be buttered. Finely chop a sprig of marjoram, savory, and a sprig of rosemary and mix them with the grated parmesan.

Remove the potatoes and porcini mushrooms from the oven and compose each flan by distributing a layer of potatoes, one of parmesan with herbs and one of porcini mushrooms in each mould, repeat the three layers and finish with the parmesan and a knob of butter; bake at 180190°C for about ten minutes. Prepare the sauce: peel the shallot, cut it in half and brown it in a saucepan with a knob of butter, a sprig of sage, a couple of bay leaves, a pinch of salt and a grind of pepper. When the shallot begins to sizzle, add 1 glass of red wine and let it evaporate; add 1 teaspoon of tomato paste and cook for 10 minutes; finally remove the aromatic herbs and blend until you obtain a smooth and homogeneous sauce. Serve the flans with the sauce; accompanied to taste with porcini mushrooms sautéed in a pan with a knob of butter.

PERCH AND TAPIOCA CUTTLET

Time 40 min

ingredients

6 people servings

6 perch fillets

300 grams of tomatoes

120 g tapioca pearls

Corn flour, egg white

tomato paste

basil salt

Peanut oil

Preparation

For the perch and tapioca cutlet recipe, cut the cherry tomatoes into small pieces and blend them.

Collect the pulp in a sieve lined with a cloth, place it on a container, and let it drain until you obtain 100 g of tomato water. Cook the tapioca in 300 g of boiling salted water. When the tapioca pearls begin to swell and become slightly transparent, add the tomato water and cook for 1520 minutes. In the meantime, bread the fish fillets, dipping in the corn flour, then in 1 beaten egg white and again in the corn flour. Fry them in hot peanut oil for 2 minutes per side. Mix the pureed tomato pulp with 1 tablespoon of concentrate, obtaining a sauce. Serve the fried fillets in the tapioca soup and complete with tomato sauce and fresh basil leaves.

CHICKEN WITH CREAM AND PORCINI

Time 45 min

ingredients

4 people

1.5kg 1 chicken

500 g of fresh cream

400 g of fresh porcini mushrooms

grappa 150 g

1 onion, garlic

butter, sage

Rosemary

parsley

extra virgin olive oil

salt and pepper

Preparation

For the chicken with cream and porcini recipe, cut the chicken into 8 pieces and brown it over high heat in a pan with 1 clove of garlic, without adding fat. Scented with some sage and rosemary leaves. Once cooked, after 45 minutes, pour in the brandy, salt and pepper. Cover with the lid and leave to cook for about 20 minutes. Chop the onion and sauté it in a large pan with a knob of butter, a drizzle of oil and a pinch of salt. Add the cream, bring it to the boil, turn off the heat and season with salt and pepper. Clean the mushrooms and cut them into small pieces.

Brown them in a pan with a drizzle of oil and 1 clove of garlic with the peel, for 23 minutes. Season with salt and pepper, then add a small, finely chopped clove of garlic. Chop half of the browned porcini mushrooms and add them to the cream. Also add the chicken, together with part of its cooking juices, and cook everything for 5 minutes over low heat, with the lid on. Finally add the remaining mushrooms and serve with fresh parsley.

PUMPKIN CHICKPEAS AND MUSHROOMS MEATLOAF,

Time 90 minutes

ingredients

4 people

1.5 kg of pumpkin

300 g of porcini mushrooms

230 g of boiled chickpeas

150 grams of spinach

2 eggs, thyme, garlic

parsley

Grated parmesan

breadcrumbs, vinegar

extra virgin olive oil

salt and pepper

Preparation

Cut the pumpkin into small pieces, remove the seeds, place them on a baking tray covered with baking paper, season with oil, thyme sprigs, salt and pepper and bake at 180°C for 1 hour. Remove from the oven and recover the pulp; cut it into pieces and blend with chickpeas, eggs, salt, pepper and 1 tablespoon of vinegar. Blanch the spinach in boiling salted water, drain and spread out on sheets of kitchen paper to dry. Clean the mushrooms and cut them into chunks; brown them in a pan with a drizzle of oil, 1 clove of garlic, salt and pepper, for 3 minutes, then complete with a sprig of chopped parsley. Spread the pumpkin mixture on a sheet of baking paper brushed with oil, using another sheet and a rolling pin, creating a rectangular base. Trim the edges and cover the rectangle of pasta with spinach. Then distribute the mushrooms on the shortest side of the rectangle and from there roll up the meatloaf using the baking paper. Mix 1 tablespoon of breadcrumbs with 1 tablespoon of grated parmesan and sprinkle the surface of the meatloaf, then bake at 170°C for about 25 minutes.

STUFFED COURGETTES

Time 80 min

ingredients

6 people

1 kg 6 courgettes

500 g of diced veal meat

50 g of raw ham

40 g of dry breadcrumbs

20 g grated parmesan

1 egg, milk

1 stalk of celery

1 carrot, 1/2 onion

parsley

dry white wine

extra virgin olive oil

salt and pepper

Preparation

For the stuffed courgettes recipe, cut the courgettes horizontally, obtaining a thicker part, the base, and a thinner part, the lid. Generously empty the thickest part and keep the pulp obtained. Blanch the bases and lids in boiling salted water for 2 minutes; Drain them on kitchen paper. Chop the celery, carrot and onion and sauté them in a large pan with 3 tablespoons of oil for 23 minutes. Add the veal pulp and brown it over a high heat, being careful not to burn the vegetables;

After 57 minutes add 1/2 glass of white wine and 1 ladle of water; lower the heat, cover and cook for about 20 minutes, then add the courgette pulp, another ladle of water, salt, pepper and cook for another 15 minutes. Finally, drain the meat (reserve the cooking juices), chop and mix it with the egg, parmesan, chopped ham, breadcrumbs soaked in milk and squeezed out, 1 tablespoon of chopped parsley, salt and pepper. Stuff the bases of the courgettes with the mixture, close with the lids and secure with a few turns of string. Place the courgettes in a baking dish, and add the cooking juices and a drop of water, if necessary. Bake at 180°C for 2025 minutes.

SEAFOOD SALAD

Time 1h

ingredients

4 people

12 peeled red prawns

12 scampi

12 medium calamari cut into pieces

4 medium potatoes, diced

1 shallot sliced

lemon, parsley

vegetable broth

extra virgin olive oil

salt and pepper

Preparation

For the seafood salad recipe, brown the shallot in a little oil, then add the potatoes, cover with the hot vegetable broth and cook until cooked: blend and season with salt and pepper. Shell prawns and scampi without removing the head; steam them for a maximum of 45 minutes and do the same with the squid. Distribute the potato cream on the plates and complete with scampi, prawns and calamari. Season with a drizzle of oil and decorate with aromatic herbs, candied lemon wedges, puffed fregola and potato chips.

VEGETABLE SKEWERS WITH OKRA

Time 45 min

ingredients

4 people

500g fresh okra

200g chilli sticks

200 g carrot sticks

100 g of breadcrumbs

30 g of shelled walnuts

4 medium cabbage leaves

1 golden apple

smoked sweet paprika

extra virgin olive oil

salt, curry

Preparation

For the recipe for vegetable skewers with okra, blanch the okra in boiling salted water for 45 minutes after it has started to boil again, then drain it in cold water, drain it and dry it gently with a cloth. Blanch the other vegetables too. Blend the breadcrumbs with 1 tablespoon of curry, 1 teaspoon of paprika, the walnuts and a couple of tablespoons of oil and salt; you will have to obtain a fairly fine mixture. Assemble 4 skewers alternating the okra, apple segments and vegetable sticks on each stick (in season you can add 200 g of white asparagus); Grease them with oil and pass them in the bread mixture. Brown the skewers in a pan on both sides until golden brown. Sprinkle it with salt just before enjoying it.

MEDITERRANEAN-STYLE COD IN AGUACHILE

TO THE

Time 20 min

ingredients

4 people

600 g of skinless cod fillet

15 g of desalted capers

10 grams of fresh coriander

5 g of fresh parsley

1 serrano type of green chili pepper

1 lime, 1 lemon

extra virgin olive oil

salt and pepper

Preparation

For the Mediterranean-style cod in aguachile recipe, prepare the aguachile sauce: blend the coriander and parsley leaves (keep a few whole ones aside to complete) with the lime juice and 1/2 lemon, a pinch of salt, 2 tablespoons of oil and the green chili pepper. Grease a non-stick pan with a drizzle of oil, drain the cod over high heat for 23 minutes on each side, then lightly salt, close with the lid and continue over low heat for another 56 minutes. Distribute the cod onto plates, complete with 1 tablespoon of capers, the aguachile sauce and, to taste, lemon or lime wedges. Top with parsley or coriander leaves. The ingredient: Serrano chili pepper is a whole green chili pepper native to Mexico. If not too spicy, it can be replaced with other similar varieties.

PORK FILLET WITH LIEGE SYRUP, FRIGGITELLI AND SPILLION ONIONS

Time 35 min

ingredients

4 people

500 g clean

Borettane onions

600 g 1 pork fillet

400 g of friggitelli peppers

thyme, bay leaf

extra virgin olive oil

salt and pepper

Preparation

For the recipe of pork fillet with Liège syrup, friggitelli and spring onions, salt and pepper

the fillet, sprinkle it with chopped thyme, and brown it on all sides in a pan with a drizzle of oil, in about 67 minutes. Add the spring onions, a couple of bay leaves, 2 tablespoons of Liège syrup, salt and pepper and cook until the fillet reaches 58°C in the centre, about 20 minutes, turning several times. During cooking the onions will release a little water, which will serve to dilute the syrup and meat juices, creating a sauce. Check evaporation during cooking and, if necessary, add a drop of water. Separately, sauté the friggitelli in another pan with a drizzle of oil for 810 minutes. Serve the roast with its sauce and onions; completed with friggitelli, the Mediterranean note in a more continental dish.

SEA BREAM AND CARAMELIZED ENDIVE

Time 1h

ingredients

4 people servings

2 sea bream, 800 g each.

4 heads of Belgian endive

honey, lemon

garlic, sage

rosemary, butter

thyme, bay leaf

Dry Marsala

extra virgin olive oil

salt and pepper

Preparation

For the sea bream and caramelized endive recipe, clean the sea bream: scale them, remove the fins and gut them; obtain 4 fillets, trimming the ventral part, which is softer and full of bones. Keep the head, midbone and belly cutouts. Brown all the fish scraps in a pan with a thin layer of oil, a sprig of rosemary, a little thyme and 1 bay leaf; after 10 minutes add 1/2 glass of dry Marsala and continue cooking for another 30 minutes, stirring occasionally; finally filter and thicken the sauce on the heat, with a small piece of butter, for 5 minutes. In a pan, heat a drizzle of oil with a sprig of rosemary, 2 sage leaves and 1 clove of garlic over medium heat; add the sea bream fillets, positioning themselves with the skin facing downwards, cover with the cover and cook for about ten minutes (the steam that forms inside will also cook the fillets on the surface). Cut the 4 endive heads in half and steam for 10 minutes. In the meantime, blend 3 tablespoons of honey with 3 tablespoons of oil and 2 lemon peels, salt and pepper and, to taste, a few chervil leaves. Transfer the endive to a baking tray, brush with the honey emulsion and bake at 200°C for 45 minutes. Serve the sea bream fillets with the sauce and accompany them with the escarole. To be recovered: the fish waste, rich in flavour, is used to prepare the sauce that accompanies the fillets.

MARENGO CHICKEN

Time 45 min

ingredients

6 people servings

1.2kg 1 chicken

500 grams of tomatoes

150 g of champignon mushrooms

6 prawn tails

6 eggs, flour, garlic,

homemade bread

chopped parsley

dry white wine

salt, butter, lemon

extra virgin olive oil

Preparation

For the chicken Marengo recipe, cut the chicken into 6 pieces, separating the breast and thighs. Flour them and brown them in a large pan with a drizzle of oil, a knob of butter and 1 clove of garlic crushed in the peel. Turn the pieces on all sides for 56 minutes. Deglaze the chicken with 1 glass of wine, then add the chopped tomatoes. Add salt and cook for 5 minutes. Remove the breasts and add the sliced mushrooms. Cook for another 10 minutes, then add the breasts again, the juice of 1/2 lemon and 2 tablespoons of parsley and finish cooking in 12 minutes. Toast 6 slices of bread. Fry the fried eggs for 5 minutes. Roast the peeled prawn tails, then add them to the sauce with the chicken. Serve the chicken in its sauce, with the egg on the bread.

CONCLUSION

"The journey of the bariatric diet is a complex and fascinating journey. This book has provided an in-depth overview of the underlying scientific principles and practical strategies for achieving your goals. Remember that long-term success depends not only on nutrition, but also by regular exercise, the support of a medical team and a profound lifestyle change. Continue to inform yourself and take care of yourself, and the results will be evident." "You have embarked on an extraordinary journey towards a new you. This book has given you the tools and motivation to face challenges and achieve your goals. Remember that you are stronger than you think and that every small step brings you closer to your goal. Celebrate your successes, be patient with yourself and continue to inspire yourself. You can transform your life!"

"I hope this book has accompanied you on this journey of discovery and personal growth. The bariatric diet is much more than just weight loss; it is an opportunity to rediscover yourself, your tastes and your passions. Remember that you are unique and that your journey is personal. Don't be afraid to experiment, ask for help and celebrate every little victory." Now you have all the information you need to embark on this new chapter in your life. Don't wait any longer! Start putting the advice in this book into practice and create a personalized meal plan that satisfies you. Keep striving, learning and growing. You are capable of achieving any goal you set yourself." Share your experience with us! Leave a review and tell us how this book helped you.

Thank you for dedicating your time and attention to these pages, for showing a sincere interest in understanding and improving your health. Your words could be a guiding light for other wellness seekers embarking on this path. I thank you deeply for choosing The Bariatric Diet 2024. Thank you very much for choosing to accompany me on this journey and for investing in your health and well-being. I wish you all the success and happiness in your future journey.With gratitude,

TERY LONG